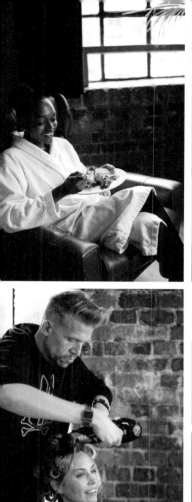
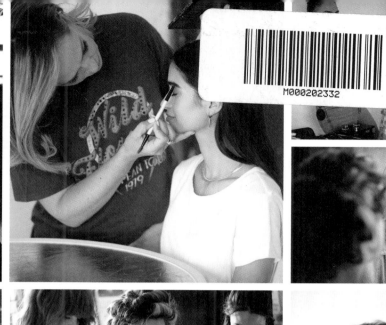
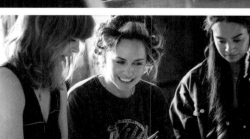
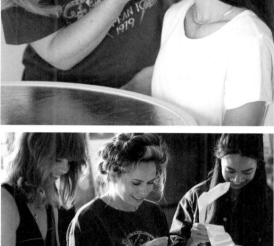
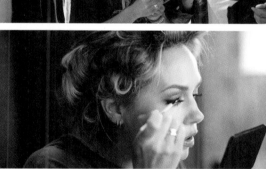
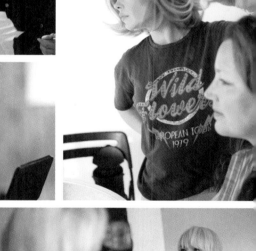
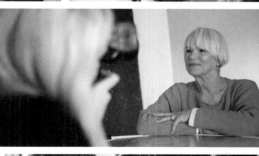
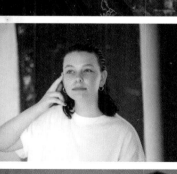
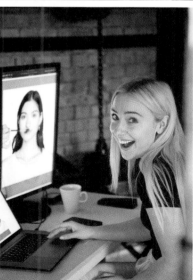
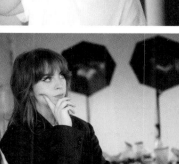

Make Up

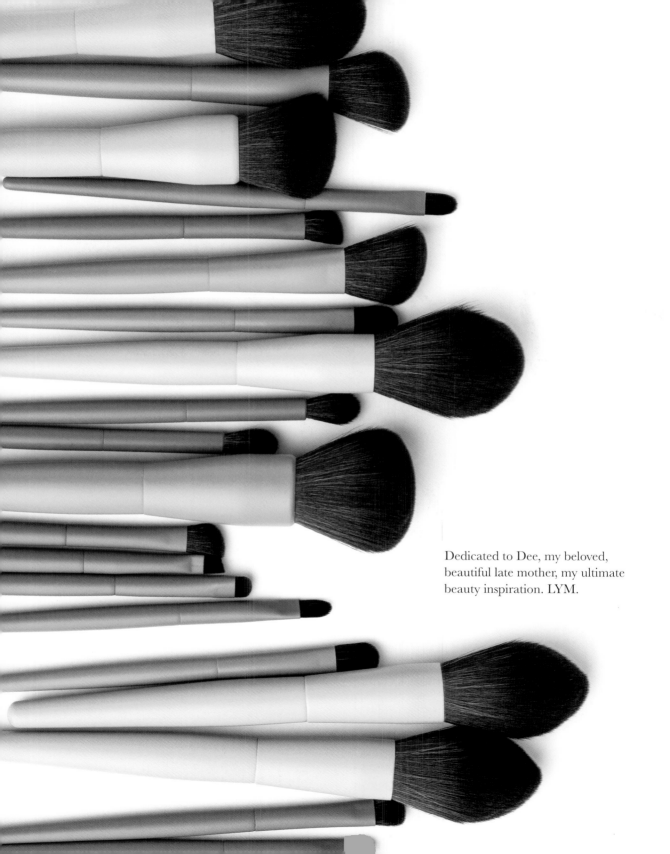

Dedicated to Dee, my beloved, beautiful late mother, my ultimate beauty inspiration. LYM.

Make Up

HANNAH MARTIN

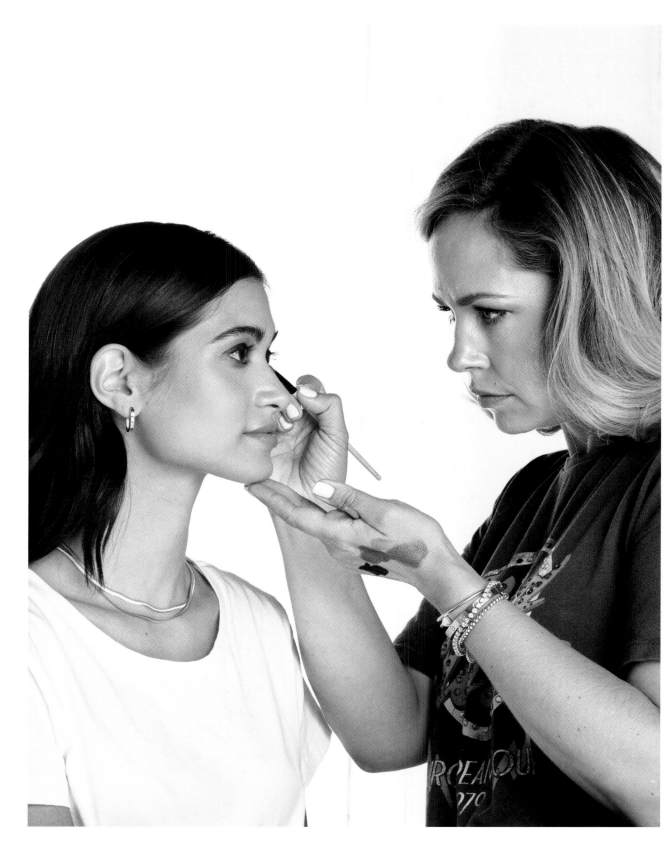

WHERE IT ALL STARTED

I can pinpoint the time I first verbalised that I wanted to be a makeup artist. I was in a session with my university counsellor. She asked me, as I sobbed miserably in the chair, what it was I really wanted to do. Through the tears, I admitted that I wanted to go to the London College of Fashion and study Theatrical Makeup. There, I'd finally said it.

I was exhausted. I was unfulfilled and joyless studying nursing. I love people, therefore I really enjoyed certain aspects of my nursing training and I learnt essential skills that I will forever be thankful for. But my spirit was being crushed with no creative outlet. I knew, deep down, that this just wasn't for me. You see, I only studied nursing because I didn't get into theatre school. I applied to the top classical schools and they all said the same thing – you're too 'commercial'. Granted, I've always had a baby-face, but I think I was a particularly young-looking 18-year-old. They advised that if I was serious about acting, that I go away and get some life experience and try again later. Well, goodness. This was a huge blow to my confidence and incredibly embarrassing as I had always assumed I'd be a thespian.

I spent my A-level year concentrating on perfecting my role of Sally Bowles in *Cabaret* for the end-of-year show and not enough time on my school work, because I was convinced I wouldn't need exam results to further my theatrical career. I was wrong. So, my initial reaction was to go to an open-call casting for the popular TV show *Hollyoaks*, knowing it was about as commercial as acting could get, and they didn't want me either! Yikes! I was thrown. I had to go back to the drawing board – with an unexpected gap year and ultimately a place at uni to study nursing.

From that very moment I verbalised my dream, I chased after a career in makeup with every ounce of energy I had. You see, I'd always loved makeup, I just never knew I could make a job out of it.

I mean, I was a total tomboy growing up, a very late bloomer, and sport was my main interest. However, in the background was a fascination with makeup and the ability to create art on a face. I'd sit at my mother's feet as she got ready at her dressing table (which I still have safe in my garage) and watch, transfixed, as she dotted her orange Vichy tinted moisturiser over her face and then blended it, the lid of an old compact mirror balanced between her fingers (I still have that too!). I'd stare intently as she lined her eyes with her favourite green Dior eyeliner pencil and curled her lashes until they were almost vertical from her lash line, then meticulously applied plenty of mascara to create the longest, featheriest lashes I'd ever seen. She'd then – and I absolutely do not recommend or condone this – painstakingly separate each lash using a nappy pin (DO NOT TRY THIS AT HOME) until her lashes were perfect.

> *I have one of my mum's mascara nappy pins stuck onto my makeup mirror with Blu Tack in front of me as I type. It holds such special memories of my favourite things: my mother and makeup!*

I've never been able to live down the tale of one time, as a tiny child, my mother had booked a session for my sister and me at a local studio to take some photos give to my dad for his birthday. On telling me we were about to leave, I ran upstairs to 'get ready' so I would look good in Daddy's photos and presented myself a few moments later having used a felt tip over my face in all the colours of the rainbow. Oh, how my mother scrubbed to get the pen off! To this day, my dad has the pictures of my sister and me in our matching outfits, basin-bowl haircuts and my beetroot-red face!

As I got older, I was gifted children's Tinkerbell makeup from the Disney store – remember the fun nail varnish that came off in the bath? This became my prized possession, even if I was jealous that my sister was given a pink set and mine was bronze (the joke's on me now, hey, with my bronzer obsession!). As a teen, I started asking for chemist vouchers for birthdays and Christmases so I could visit their makeup section and select bits from their younger collections – you know, the tea tree oil spot treatment, the concealer, the clear gloss, the clear mascara (which I remember keeping in my pencil case in an attempt to be cool!).

Then, when my sister and I were in our early teens, our mum booked herself an appointment at the Clinique counter in the nearest town for a makeup lesson. That was the day that I realised the truly transformative power of makeup. Yes, my mum was absolutely beautiful but when she got home wearing her new makeup, I literally couldn't believe my eyes. The green eyeliner was gone, replaced with a soft, shimmering champagne shadow with a neutral brown eyeliner. Her coral blush had been replaced by a soft, browny-pink (bring back Mocha Pink!) and her deep berry, oh so 90s, lip colour was now a moist, glistening, neutral lip tone – she looked RADIANT. Pretty. Feminine. Confident. She was sparkling from her updated look AND from the time, care and attention given to her by the consultant.

▌ *Whatever this magic was, I wanted in!*

I started wearing makeup myself not long after that moment. When I was about 14, there was one evening at a youth group that my sister and I went to when one of the leaders said, 'Gosh Hannah, I've never seen you in proper makeup, you look lovely'. That was another key moment for me.

I absolutely loved the process of getting ready and applying makeup and I seemed to have a natural flair for it. I always was better at art than writing essays, so there started the next phase of my makeup fascination: doing my own, doing my friends, doing my mum's.

At uni, I bunked off lectures one day with my friend Holly as she was having an Andy Warhol-inspired picture made of herself for her twenty-first birthday, so we spent the day at my house creating lots of different looks. We did a 50s movie star red-lip look with big curly hair; a Catherine Zeta-Jones-inspired green smoky eye with straight hair and a pinky Barbie look, which turned into an intense-pink smoky eye. It's no surprise, looking back, that this day was one of my favourite uni memories.

From that weeping counselling session, I went to speak to my tutors to say that I'd finish the last year of my course, but I wouldn't do my dissertation or the management module, so I had to settle for a diploma rather than a degree. Not a problem. I was excited to get started on the next phase of my life and I didn't even go to my graduation! Instead, I got a part-time job at the Benefit counter, by far the coolest counter Debenhams Oxford had at the time. Dedicated and loving it, I swiftly, kind of by accident, went from being the weekend girl to working part-time, to working full time, to becoming the Account Manager (thank you, Mel, for the opportunity). It was here that I not only got to practise applying makeup to customers, I learnt about life in retail, pitching, selling, teamwork, business and so much more. I absolutely loved my time and the people from those days. Lots of us are all still in touch thanks to social media. I was there for just over a year, but left Oxford after I got married, so young at just 23, and I moved to London to pursue a career in makeup.

I was convinced that I'd quickly settle into London life and carve out a career as a makeup artist, but I really had no idea what I was entering into. A good example of this was when I arranged to assist a photographer, David Jones, for Fashion Week. A brilliant gig, I thought. It would get me in front of loads of makeup artists, who I could give my handmade business cards to and I would make tonnes of connections. Well, day one I realised it wouldn't be so easy. Firstly, I stood out like a sore thumb as I rocked up at the tents at the Natural History Museum in my favourite sparkly, multicoloured Mango blouse – I clearly hadn't got the all-black everything memo – and I spent my time racing from venue to venue, marking up the photographer's spot at the end of the catwalk (the bonus of being small, I suppose), not mingling backstage with the MUAs as I'd expected. I looked like I didn't know what I was doing and the truth was, I really didn't.

After a few months assisting, doing test shoots with my teeny-tiny kit case and not earning a penny, my sweet husband begged me to get a job. His words were, 'I love that you're trying, babe, but I think we need you to be paid just for a year or so while we get started.' He was absolutely right. We were spending every penny of my husband Simon's salary on rent and living costs – I had no idea renting in London would be so expensive – not to mention the travel costs, etc., and we didn't have a penny spare. It was tight, tight, tight.

So, back to retail I went. Initially, I worked for Clinique in Fenwick Bond Street. I loved the store. I loved Mayfair, but I rarely did any makeup despite offering everyone who approached the counter. I'd stand gazing adoringly at the Bobbi Brown counter opposite me. There was no Bobbi Brown where I grew up, so the only times I ever got to see the products were on my makeup shopping trips to London that my friend Holly and I would take. Their artists always looked wonderful and they did makeup on customers all day, every day. I was in awe.

I took it upon myself to call the Area Manager for Bobbi Brown to enquire about a job. I was desperate to work for the woman whose products I loved and whose books I'd read in Blackwell's. I'm not ashamed to say I called her every day for 2 weeks until she agreed to meet me at a local coffee shop. She gave me a job, and what was supposed to be a year's job in order to be salaried, to be able to use the discount to build up my kit and practise makeup on different faces, became a 12-year career.

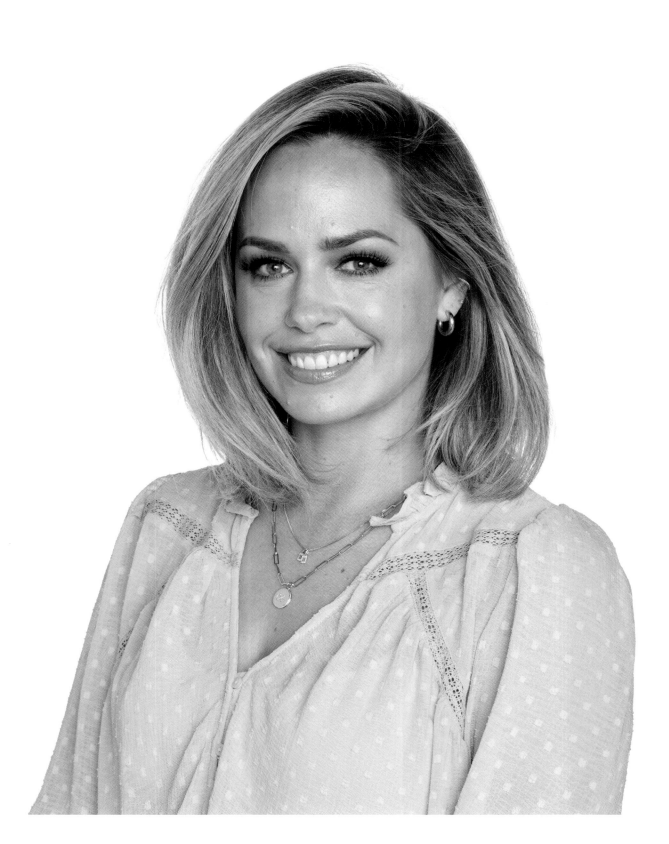

I ultimately became the Artistry Manager for the brand in the UK and Ireland, working as part of the Global Leadership Team and in Bobbi's elite team of artists!

I could never have predicted that was going to happen, but I'm so glad it did. In working for the brand, I spent 3 years as a manager for two counters, then I got the role of Pro Artist, travelling the country doing events and press for the brand, then becoming senior Pro and finally Artistry Manager, all the while being used by the press office for major events. These included getting celebrities ready for the red carpet, TV appearances, beauty shoots, stints on breakfast television, working London and New York Fashion Weeks, not to mention trips to New York for product development meetings, and to China to teach their artists and lead events (the stories I could tell . . .). I was working with designers, high-profile brides, writing magazine features and contributing to books – the opportunities were varied and plentiful. And all this came before social media!

I really did have the time of my life, but there came a point, after Bobbi herself left, that I realised I too needed to spread my wings to further my career. It was whilst I was on maternity leave with my daughter (a sibling for my son – my miracle baby after years of trying, fertility treatment and loss) that I spoke with my dear friend and mentor Krishna, and decided to take the leap of faith and start my freelance career.

It's been a wild time and the best move I could have possibly made. I've had to learn and grow so much as a person and as a makeup artist. My career is so varied – from beauty shoots to shoots with personal clients, brand collaborations, brand ambassadorships, TV work, consultancy, teaching at a makeup school, content creation for social media and so on, and I love it all! Honestly, every day I count myself lucky that I work in a field I adore. I still get the same butterflies opening press packages now that I did when sitting on the bus on the way home from town, opening the new Juicy Tube I'd been saving for.

I have learnt so much in the last 17 years or so about makeup: how to apply it, how to manipulate skin and product to get the finish you want – the short cuts you can take, the ones you absolutely can't – and I intend to pour it all into these pages, so you too can feel knowledgeable and empowered with your makeup. I'm not the best makeup artist out there – I've made a tonne of mistakes along the way – but I do love sharing what I know and nothing gives me more joy than helping others feel good about themselves.

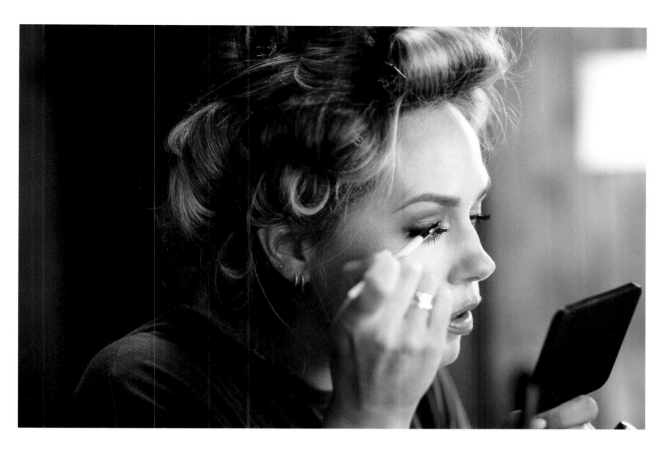

> *Makeup is not essential. No one needs it, but makeup and the art of applying it can be incredibly powerful, therapeutic even, an act of self-love to boost your wellbeing.*

This has become known in the industry as the 'Lipstick Effect', a phrase first coined by Leonard Lauder of Estee Lauder Companies when, after the atrocities of 9/11, the sales of lipstick increased. This was also seen during periods of economic crisis and the stresses of the pandemic.

I'm far more concerned with how makeup makes you **feel** than how it makes you **look**. I hope that within these pages I give you the tools, knowledge and confidence to help you look and feel your very best.

Hannah

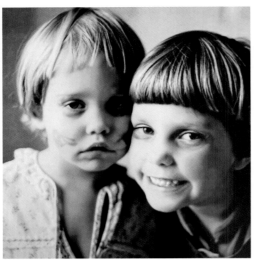

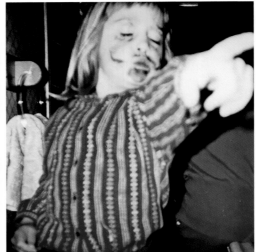

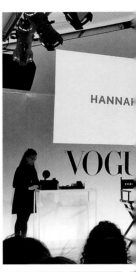

HANNAH

VOGU

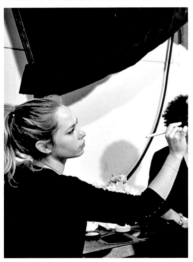

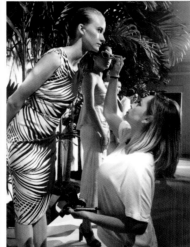

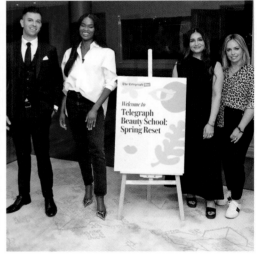

Welcome to
Telegraph
Beauty School:
Spring Reset

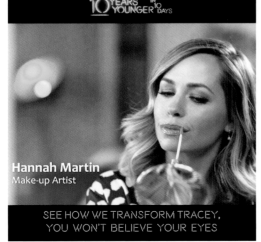

10 YEARS YOUNGER IN 10 DAYS

Hannah Martin
Make-up Artist

SEE HOW WE TRANSFORM TRACEY,
YOU WON'T BELIEVE YOUR EYES

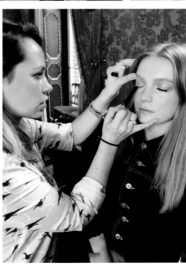

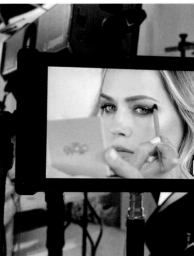

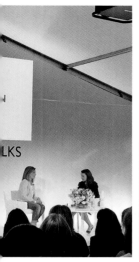
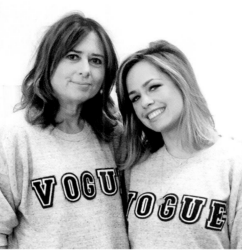
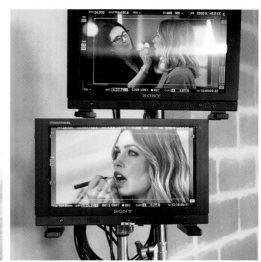
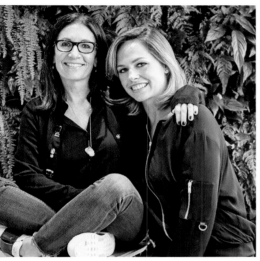
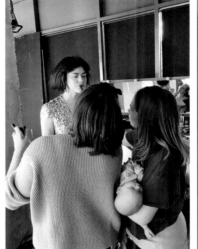
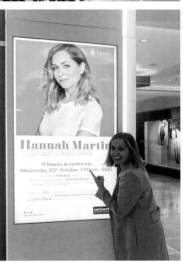
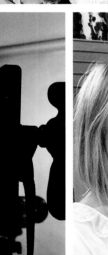
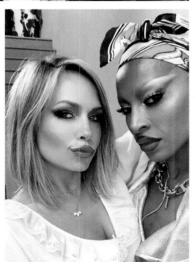
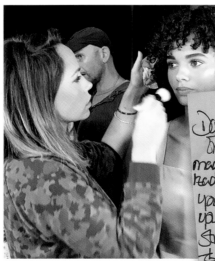
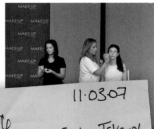

11·03·07

Dave
Enclosed from Sunday Telegraph
mag (that I don't usually
read!) It's just to encourage
you not to lose sight of
your dream. Sounds up your
street my love so will continue
to pray for an opening. Lys.
M.irimana

SKIN PREP

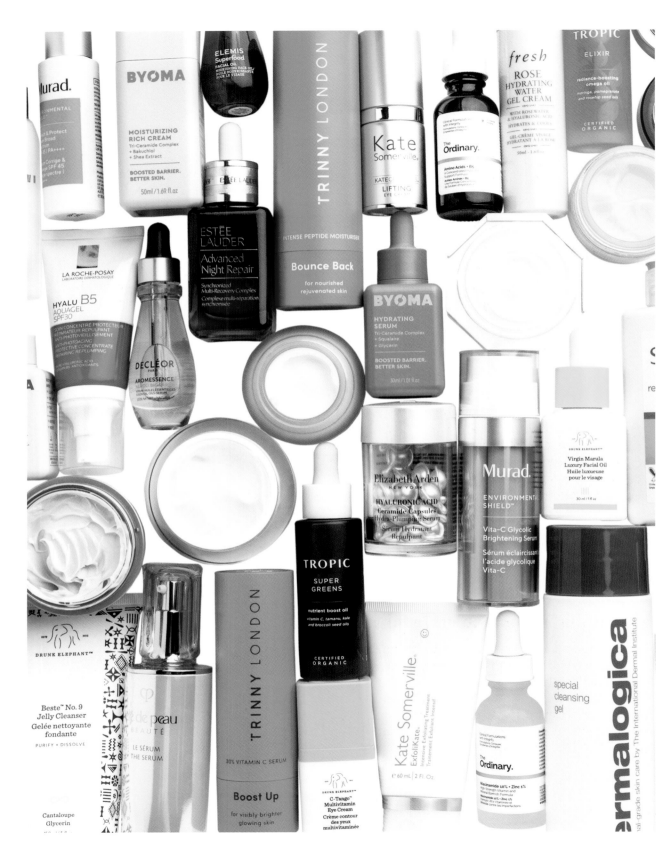

SKIN PREP

I often come across the assumption that foundation is the key to perfecting a skin look when, truthfully, it's all about how you prep your skin for makeup, i.e. skincare.

> *Some makeup lovers prefer to invest in makeup rather than their skincare items, or at least don't appreciate the importance of the products beneath their makeup. However, ultimately these have the greatest impact on how your base makeup looks and feels.*

I heard an analogy from my dear friend Zara, which really helps explain this. Think of a cake. You want to make the best cake you've ever tasted. You don't have all the ingredients that you need for the sponge, but you're not worried because you know your icing is the best going, made with the finest ingredients money can buy. So, you mix together the bits you do have – some flour, an egg, some baking powder – and hope for the best. Are you going to get a light, fluffy sponge from a cake batter with no butter or sugar and only one egg? No! No amount of delicious icing is going to make that a good cake. It's the same with makeup. If you don't prepare your skin for makeup using skincare products suitable for its needs, even the best foundation isn't going to make your skin look good.

USING SKINCARE TO PERFECT YOUR FOUNDATION

You can use skincare to manipulate how a foundation looks on the skin. If you want your makeup to be more matte in finish, then use less skincare and opt for light, water-based serums and moisturisers. If you prefer more of a dewy finish, then use skincare that's a bit richer and emollient-based, so the surface layer of your skin is saturated with hydration. This means your foundation will mix with the topical skincare and create more of a glow.

*

Topical skincare:
This is skincare applied onto the surface of the skin. For example, foundation will mix with whatever moisturiser or other skincare might already be sitting on the surface of the skin.

Matte finish:
This is when your base makeup doesn't have any shine to it and therefore looks more velvety in finish.

Dewy finish:
This is when your skincare and makeup combine and leave the skin with a healthy glow, a shine that looks like youthful, healthy, well-hydrated skin. There is none of the unwanted shine that you might get in the T-zone if you have oily skin.

A Winning Skin Prep Routine

A comprehensive skin prep routine doesn't need to be expensive, thankfully, but it may take 2 minutes to apply before you can get cracking with your base. Trust me, it's time well spent.

For anyone reading this and thinking you really don't need much skincare before makeup, bear with me. It's taken nearly 20 years of painting people's faces to come to this preferred routine. I swear by lots of light layers to achieve a brilliantly prepped skin, much like I believe in light layers of makeup to create natural, flawless, but long-wearing makeup.

This is, of course, a generic routine that can be tweaked for each individual's skin needs. I'm also writing here as a makeup artist, not a skin expert, so for specialist advice do look elsewhere. However, broadly speaking, these are the steps I recommend:

1 **Cleanser**   5 **Serum**

2 **Essence**   6 **Moisturiser**

3 **Eye cream**   7 **SPF**

4 **Lip balm**

Cleanser

I suggest you start the day with a light cleanse using a **water-based cleanser**. A light gel wash like the Simple Refreshing Facial Wash is a lovely way to wake up and its job is to break down any perspiration and oil that the skin will have produced overnight. It also cleans the skin of any remnants of the skincare used the night before.

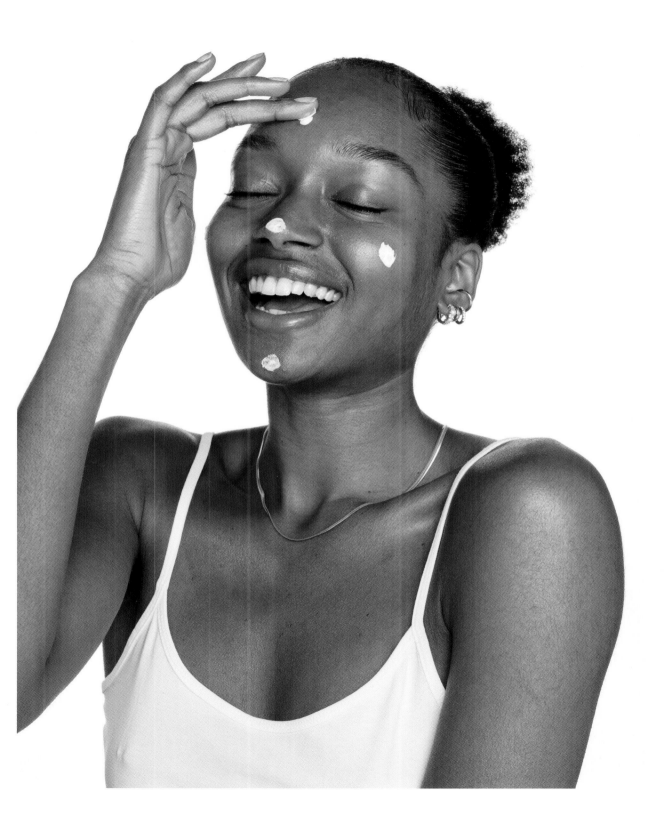

In the evening I recommend using an eye makeup remover to remove any eye makeup before I double cleanse – first with a balm and then with a cream.

Most water-based face washes are best applied to damp skin. Massage over the face and neck and then rinse using a damp flannel. Oils and balms are best applied to dry skin first, with water added once you have massaged them into the skin. Warm water typically makes oil and balms emulsify and become milky in texture. Continue to massage for a few moments, then rinse with a damp flannel.

Some cream cleansers stipulate that they're best removed with a cotton pad. Thankfully, there are now lots of reusable and machine-washable cotton pads available to buy. If you use a cream cleanser in the morning – and you may wish to if your skin is very dry – be sure to follow with a toner to remove any residual cleanser left on the skin.

Exfoliate:
This will remove dead skin cells from the surface of the skin using a granular substance, a chemical or an exfoliation tool, and it will encourage skin cell turnover.

Super sheer:
Very light makeup coverage.

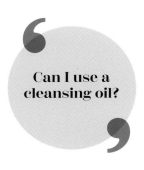

Can I use a cleansing oil?

I'm obsessed with cleansing oils and have been for years, but I tend to keep these for makeup removal rather than makeup prep as I don't want to add any unwanted oil to the skin before makeup. I believe oil to be one of the very best makeup removers, but it's not necessary first thing in the morning. A lighter, water-based cleanser will do just fine.

CLEANSERS I LIKE:

Balms
- Elemis Pro-Collagen Cleansing Balm
- Pixi Double Cleanse
- Augustinus Bader The Cleansing Balm
- Beauty Pie Japanfusion
- Clinique Take The Day Off Cleansing Balm

Washes
- CeraVe Hydrating Cleanser
- La Roche-Posay Toleriane Softening Foaming Gel
- Elemis Superfood Facial Wash
- Skingredients Sally Cleanse (for blemish-prone skin)

Oils
- Bobbi Brown Soothing Cleansing Oil
- Elemis Superfood Facial Oil
- Erborian Centella Cleansing Oil
- Clarins Total Cleansing Oil
- Kora Organics Milky Mushroom Gentle Cleansing Oil

Scrubs
- Dermalogica Daily Microfoliant
- Frank Body Original Face Scrub
- Fresh Sugar Strawberry Exfoliating Face Wash
- La Roche-Posay Ultrafine Scrub
- Avène Gentle Exfoliating Gel

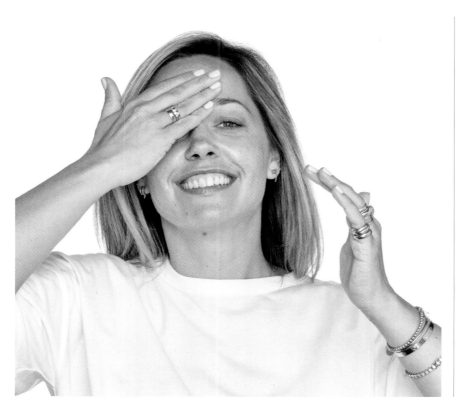

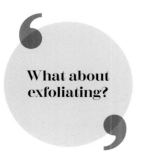

What about exfoliating?

Exfoliating is key to prepping skin before makeup, but I prefer to do this in the evening before bed so I can immediately moisturise and allow my skin to settle overnight. I usually advise my clients to exfoliate the night before a big makeup moment with a gentle scrub rather than an acid, as this will gently remove any dry dead skin cells with no risk of burning the skin.

Sometimes clients go heavy on the retinol the night before an event in the hope of creating a fresh base for makeup the next day. Whilst you can't see the effect of overdoing the acids on makeup-free skin, you can tell as soon as you try to apply any makeup. The skin can have a very fine, crepey texture, which makeup gets caught in no matter how much you moisturise or try to treat the skin with oils. I once had a bridesmaid who had had a chemical peel the week of the wedding and even the lightest tinted moisturiser was showing texture on the skin. I eventually had to take the makeup off, reapply skincare and use powder makeup. I know it doesn't make sense, but the powder foundation actually looked much less obvious on the skin.

A Quick Fix for Dry or Flaky Skin Patches

If you ever find yourself in a situation where you want to do your makeup and have an area of dry or flaky skin, don't panic – all you need is a face oil and a cotton bud (or Q-tip for my friends overseas!).

Let's take dry skin around the nose as an example (but I've frequently come across it on the chin and between the brows too). If your makeup is clinging to the dry skin, take some face oil (moisturiser will also work but I find oil much more effective for this remedy) and massage it into the area. Let it sink in for a few minutes, then use a cotton bud to gently massage it in using small circular motions. You should start to see the little flakes of skin soften as they become saturated in oil and come away on the cotton bud. Once you've done that and cleaned off any excess oil with something like a micellar water, you will be able to reapply the makeup and it will sit smoothly on the skin.

Essence

> *A lot of people assume an essence is an unnecessary step in skin prep and it's just beauty brands wanting us to part with more cash. But it's a total game changer!*

Time for another analogy: imagine a kitchen sponge (glamorous). Now, think about adding a drop of washing-up liquid to that sponge. When it's dry, the washing-up liquid will just sit on the surface of the sponge and it won't be absorbed or start foaming. Add the same drop of washing-up liquid to a wet sponge and, wahey, you're off – it will bubble easily and you're ready to get your dishes all clean. It's the same with the skin.

FACE OILS I LIKE:

– Kora Organics
  Noni Glow

– Willowberry
  Nutrient Boost
  Face Oil

– Clarins Blue Orchid
  Treatment Oil

– Drunk Elephant
  Virgin Marula
  Luxury Facial Oil

– Elizabeth Arden
  Eight Hour All-Over
  Miracle Oil

– Elemis Superfood
  Facial Oil

– Sarah Chapman
  Skinesis: Skinesis
  Overnight Facial
  Night Elixir and
  Skinesis Morning
  Facial Day Elixir

Hyaluronic acid:
This is a humectant capable of binding 1,000 times its weight in water. It is produced naturally by the body and found in the skin, eyes and synovial fluid of the joints. This acid is widely used in skincare and in makeup as a moisturiser.

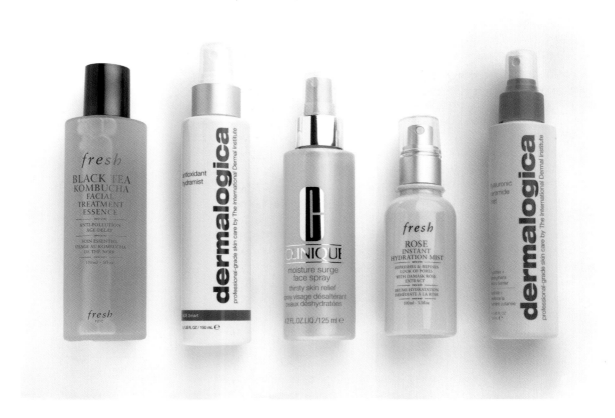

If you try to apply your moisturiser to dry skin, the moisturiser can sit on the surface of the skin and will have a harder time being absorbed. 'Wet' the skin first with an essence and your serums and moisturisers will be absorbed much more effectively. In turn, you'll also end up using less moisturiser.

Essences are essentially waters infused with, most commonly, hyaluronic acid – otherwise known as moisturiser – and glycerin, which is a humectant that helps bind moisture to the skin. So, think of essences as the first step in your moisturising routine.

To apply, shake a few drops into the palm of your hand, rub your hands together and press gently into the skin using a cupping motion with your hands. Use on your cheeks, chin, forehead and neck.

ESSENCES I LIKE:

– Bioeffect EGF Essence

– Shiseido Treatment Softener

– Clé De Peau Beauté Hydro-Softening Lotion

– La Mer The Treatment Lotion

– Fresh Kombucha Facial Treatment Essence

Eye cream

After essence (any sceptics, please trust me, it makes all the difference), I suggest it's time for a light eye cream. I'm often asked if it's really necessary to use a separate eye cream to your face cream and I really believe that it is. The skin is so much finer around the eyes and your day cream may well be too heavy and actually add to the puffiness that many of us are trying to reduce. So, yes, a lightweight eye cream is essential.

Smooth, don't drag, a grain-of-rice amount of eye cream around the eye socket or orbital bone (under the eye and under the eyebrow). This will help to plump up any fine lines and help reduce the appearance of dark circles. Yes, the effect here is subtle, but the more hydrated the skin around the eye is, the plumper it is, and therefore the further away it is from the veins and capillaries under the skin that cause the darkness. (Concealer is the one for the win here if dark circles are your concern . . . but more on that on page 227.)

Eye cream will also prep your skin for concealer, so don't overdo it, as lovely as it might feel, because it will cause your concealer to crease – save adding a good-sized dollop and saturating the skin until the evening.

On this note, if you are someone who struggles with your eyeshadow creasing, even long-wear cream shadow, then don't put any eye cream on the brow bone before makeup application, stick to just doing this in your evening routine. As eye cream is absorbed, it travels down the lid and can cause your makeup to crease. If you're this person, you may want to refrain from using foundation or concealer on your lids for the same reason. If it is an area of concern for you, I suggest using a richer, treatment eye cream at night and a lighter one before makeup to help prevent any concealer creasing.

Lip balm

I tend to do lip balm at this stage with my clients to give it time to sink in and to prep the lips before any lipstick I might apply later. I know a lot of my friends don't consider lip balm as part of their skincare routine, regarding it as more of a 'quick fix' product to keep in their handbag in case their lips get dry, but I absolutely do.

Your lips need moisture just like the rest of your face. There's also something so soothing and comforting about the texture of balm on the lips that makes your mouth feel comfortable as you prep your face.

EYE CREAMS I LIKE:

– Estée Lauder Advanced Night Repair

– Shiseido Ultimune Power Infusing Concentrate

– Shiseido Benefiance Wrinkle Smoothing Eye Cream

– Clarins Double Serum Eye

– The INKEY List Caffeine Eye Serum

– StriVectin Multi-Action R&R Eye Cream

– La Mer The Eye Concentrate

– Clinique All About Eyes

– Willowberry Reviving Eye Cream

– Bobbi Brown Vitamin Enriched Eye Base

– CeraVe Eye Repair Cream

– Elizabeth Arden Ceramide Lift and Firm Eye Cream

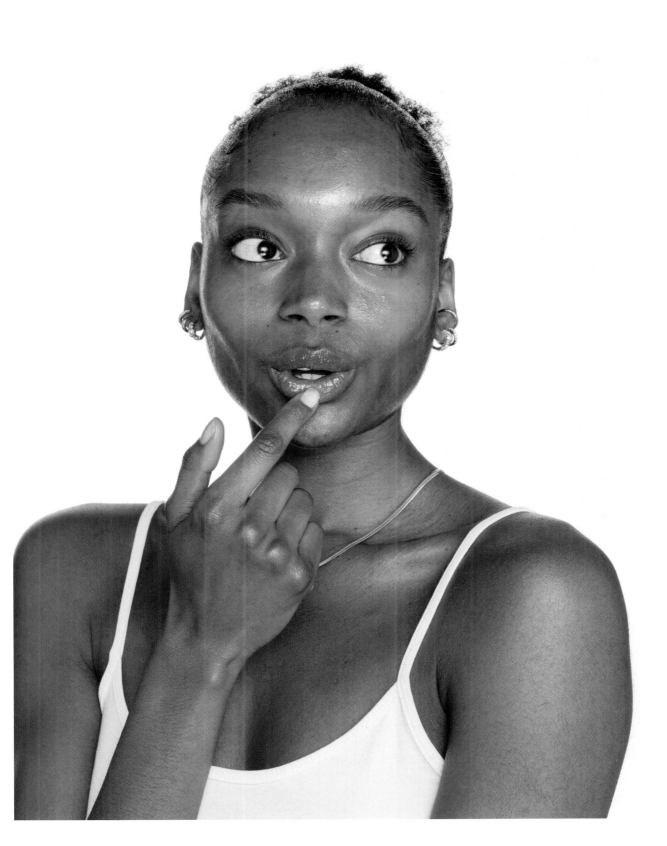

I tend to use balms that have a fairly thick texture as I prefer them for both moisturising and protection. If the lip treatment is too thin, I find the lips absorb the product really quickly and the skin doesn't feel as plump or conditioned when it comes to applying colour.

I know many don't like the sensation of having 'sticky lips', so in that case a lightweight lip balm is fine, but personally, I find the efficacy and overall finish of a slightly tackier balm really helpful. If your lips are feeling really dry and you're suffering with some flaky skin, it's best to gently exfoliate the lips and remove the dead skin cells or your lip products will stick between the flakes and won't sit smoothly.

Balms will soften the skin, so it may be that you can just wipe the flakes off with a tissue after a few minutes, but you may need the help of a lip scrub. Lip scrubs are readily available or you can easily make one at home if you don't have anything to hand. Remove with a flannel or tissue and follow with lip balm – your lips will feel so incredibly soft! Love it.

LIP BALMS I LIKE:

– Bobbi Brown Balm

– Clinique Moisture Surge Lip Hydro-Plump Treatment

– By Terry Baume de Rose

– Elizabeth Arden 8 Hour Cream Skin Protectant

– Carmex

– Dr Pawpaw Multipurpose Soothing Balm

– Bloom and Blossom Lip Service

– Ciaté Disco Nap

– Summer Fridays Lip Butter Balm

– Huda Beauty Silk Balm

A HOMEMADE LIP SCRUB

I make my lip scrub with coconut oil, honey and sugar (see page 170). The granulated sugar will gently buff away the skin cells while the honey and oil moisturise and condition your lips.

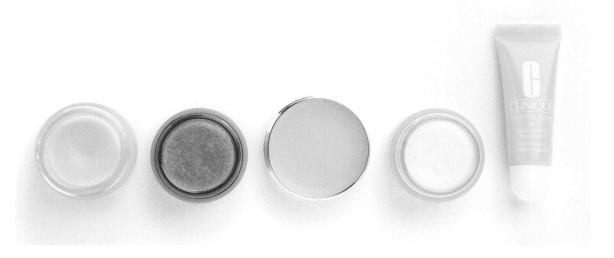

Serum

Now, time for serum. Some may skip their treatment serum in the morning and prefer to use it at night when the skin does most of its rejuvenating, but I love to use a light, hydrating serum before I progress to moisturiser, usually something water-based and pumped full of moisture-boosters, like hyaluronic acid, niacinamide, sodium hyaluronate and glycerin.

> *A serum is also a great way of feeding your skin with vitamins and antioxidants.*

Generally speaking, serums have a much thinner texture than moisturisers, meaning all the ingredients can be more effectively absorbed by the skin.

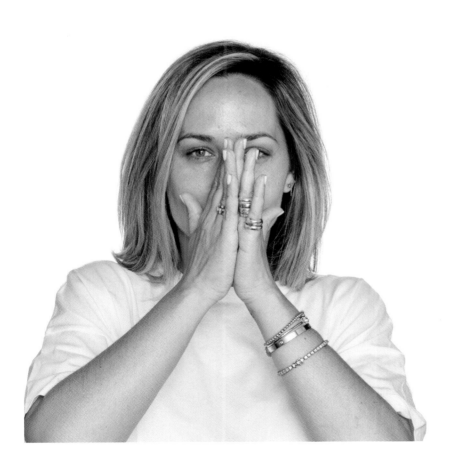

*

Niacinamide:
A form of vitamin B3 that helps build proteins in the skin and protects against environmental damage.

Glycerin:
A humectant that helps bind moisture to the skin.

Inflammation:
Skin may turn red or appear irritated.

Salicylic acid:
A beta hydroxy acid (BHA) thought to reduce acne by exfoliating the skin and dissolving the dead skin cells that may clog pores.

Lactic acid:
An alpha hydroxy acid (AHA) used to remove dead skin cells, help fade dark spots and soften fine lines.

Glycolic acid:
An alpha hydroxy acid (AHA) and a humectant used for exfoliating the skin.

Yes, nutrition is key when it comes to skin health, i.e. eating well and drinking lots of water – supporting your skin from the inside out – but you can also benefit hugely from nourishing your skin topically. This is much like the liquid feed sprayed onto the leaves and roots of tomato plants to help them grow (gosh, that's such a vivid childhood memory of helping my grandpa feed his precious plants in the greenhouse … the smell … I digress). Feeding your skin topically with serums helps in much the same way.

If dullness is your key concern, then you may prefer a vitamin C serum, of which there are many, thankfully, as vitamin C is renowned for making the skin glow and creating healthy luminosity. It's a really powerful antioxidant that neutralises the free radicals that cause skin damage, but it also blocks the enzyme responsible for melanin production, preventing the appearance of dark spots. Just be sure to use a strong daily SPF when you've used vitamin C.

If clarity is your key concern or you struggle with breakouts, then you want to look for serums that contain ingredients like salicylic acid, lactic acid and glycolic acid, all of which slough away any dead skin cells that could be blocking the pores and help reduce inflammation.

SERUMS I LIKE:

Moisturising:
– Vichy Minéral 89
– La Roche-Posay Hyalu B5 Hyaluronic Acid Serum
– CeraVe Hyaluronic Acid Serum
– Loreal Revitalift Hyaluronic Acid Serum

Vitamin C:
– Dr Dennis Gross C+Collagen
– La Roche-Posay Pure Vitamin C10
– Drunk Elephant C-Firma Fresh Day Serum

For acne-prone skin:
Look for salicylic acid and glycolic acid

– La Roche-Posay Effaclar Serum
– The Ordinary Niacinamide 10% + Zinc 1%
– Paula's Choice Skin Perfecting 2% BHA Liquid Exfoliant

RETINOL

Retinol is a form of vitamin A, used for its anti-ageing properties and to help clear acne.

Retinols I like:
· La Roche-Posay Retinol B3

· Skin Rocks Retinoid 1 and 2
· The Ordinary Retinol 0.2% in Squalane (they also have 0.5%, 1% and 2%, so excellent as a starting point as you need to build up your tolerance)
· The INKEY List Retinol Serum
· Beauty Pie Super Retinol High Dose Booster

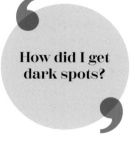

How did I get dark spots?

Dark spots are a classic symptom of sun damage, where the sun's harmful rays have damaged the 'melanocyte'. These are the cells in the basal layer of the epidermis (skin) where melanin is made. When they are damaged they can over produce melanin, resulting in dark spots and pigmentation.

Moisturiser

Once you've allowed your serum to sink in, it's time for your moisturiser. Which moisturiser you choose can significantly alter the appearance of your base makeup, so be sure to take this into consideration. Now, what do I mean by that?

If you want a really matte-looking finish from your foundation, for example, but use a heavy, oil-rich moisturiser underneath, like Weleda Skin Food, then the emollients in the moisturiser will mix with the foundation and you will create more of a glow.

In the same way, if you want a dewy look from your base makeup but use a lightweight, water-based moisturiser and your skin is more on the dehydrated side, you may not achieve the level of glow you're looking for.

> *So really, when I'm working, it's the skincare I use on my model that dictates the look of her skin more than the foundation. This often causes some confusion, because I think most people look to the foundation itself for the finish.*

Emollients:
This is a moisturising treatment that is applied to the skin to soothe and hydrate. It covers the skin with a protective film to lock in moisture.

_____

Sebum:
This waxy oil is produced by the sebaceous glands in the skin to moisturise and protect the skin.

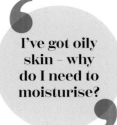

I've got oily skin – why do I need to moisturise?

I've met lots of people during my career who have been so concerned about oil and shine that in their quest for a matte look they have accidentally caused their skin to produce excess oil. This happens when the skin is starved of the necessary oil it needs to create a protective barrier in its very surface layer.

You see, all skin types need a healthy balance of water and oil in the surface layer to keep it plump and protected. But when you constantly strip the skin of its natural oils, say with harsh soaps and cleansers, and then don't replace that needed oil, your skin will panic and produce more. Then you strip it again, it produces more, and so on and so on. If you nourish your skin with the moisture it needs – granted, not too much – that cycle of overproduction is broken and you'll find, in time, that your sebum production calms down. I remember being at an Ariel Tejada masterclass, his first in the UK, and he said that was his greatest lesson when he visited a dermatologist about his skin. His skin was oily but severely dehydrated, and adding a moisturiser to his routine changed everything.

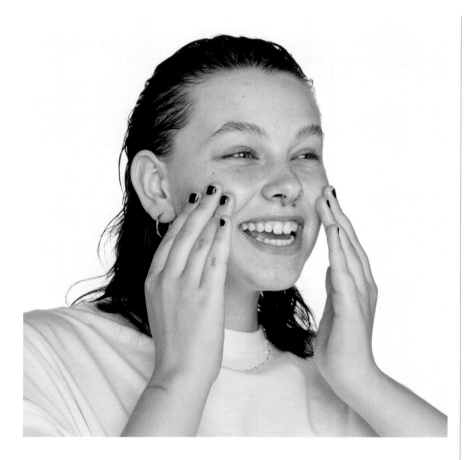

· **If you have normal, well-balanced skin**, and by that I mean not dry and not oily, a **classic day cream** will work wonders.

· **If your skin secretes a bit more oil and can look overly shiny**, I'd suggest looking for a **lightweight, water-based moisturiser**, but absolutely do moisturise.

· **If you want your foundation to look matte** then yes, look for an **oil-free, long-wearing foundation**, but also use a lightweight moisturiser underneath so as not to add too much oil to your skin.

· **If you want a more luminous finish**, do use **a richer moisturiser** as well as looking for foundations that claim to have a more dewy finish. Just be mindful that what you do before the makeup itself will have an effect on whatever product you use on top.

LIGHTWEIGHT MOISTURISERS I LIKE:

– CeraVe Facial Moisturising Lotion

– By Terry Hyaluronic Global Face Cream

– Honest Beauty Hydrogel Cream

– Bobbi Brown Hydrating Water Fresh Cream

– Clinique Moisture Surge

– Mario Badescu Oil Free Moisturiser

– Kate Somerville Oil Free Moisturiser

RICHER MOISTURISERS I LIKE:

– Charlotte Tilbury Magic Cream

– La Mer Moisturising Cream

– Bobbi Brown Vitamin Enriched Face Base

– It Cosmetics Confidence in a Cream

– Weleda Skin Food

– Kiehl's Ultra Facial Cream

– Shiseido Benefiance Wrinkle Smoothing Cream

SPF

Sunscreen should be applied daily after your moisturiser, not just when you're heading out into the sun.

I know there's some controversy about SPF and people wearing too much these days and not getting enough vitamin D, but if the sunlight is bright enough to be able to read, there's enough sunlight to cause skin damage.

USE MORE SPF THAN YOU THINK YOU NEED

Dermatologists suggest about a teaspoon amount of SPF is necessary for the face. It sounds like a lot and looks like a lot when you first start to rub it in, but trust me, it's the best thing you can do if you're wanting to prevent issues like pigmentation, fine lines and wrinkles.

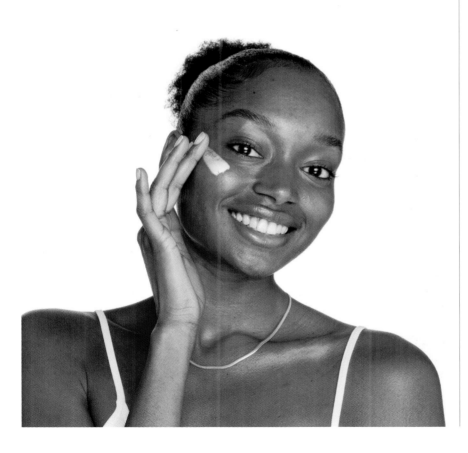

SPF FOR NORMAL SKIN:

- La Roche-Posay Anthelios UVMUNE 400 SPF 50

- Charlotte Tilbury Invisible UV Flawless Poreless Primer SPF 50

- Sun Bum Face 50 (also love their factor 50 spray for top-ups)

- Black Girl Sunscreen SPF 30

- Hello Sunday The Everyday One SPF 50

- Murad City Skin Age Defense SPF 50

- Supergoop Unseen Sunscreen SPF 30

SPF FOR OILY SKIN:

- Shiseido Urban Environment Age Defense Oil-Free SPF 30

- Beauty Pie Featherlight UVA/UVB SPF 50

- Clinique Superdefense City Block SPF 50

- Hello Sunday The Matte One SPF 50

- Kiehl's Ultra Light Daily UV Defense Aqua Gel SPF 50

- **UVA rays are present in all daylight.** They can pass through windows, so SPF is advised even when you're inside. If your desk is by a window or you spend a lot of time in the car, then you still need to safeguard your skin from the sun's damaging rays as they are the main cause of premature skin ageing.
- **UVB rays are the ones that are present in direct sunshine.**

Sun creams come in lots of different textures, so there's something to meet all skin types and needs. The key is to use enough of it. So, if a sunscreen says it is SPF 50 but you only use a tiny bit, you won't be getting the full SPF 50 protection that you think you are.

- If you have **oily skin** you might prefer a **lighter gel-based formula**.
- If you have **drier skin** like me, then something **more moisturising** will be better.

You can also choose between a physical SPF or a chemical one:

- Physical SPFs create a barrier that protects the skin. Often it's titanium dioxide or zinc oxide that's used.

SPF SPRAYS:

– Sun Bum Original SPF 50

– Kate Somerville UncompliKated SPF 50

– Clarins Sun Care Water Mist SPF 50+

– La Roche-Posay Anthelios UVMUNE 400 SPF 50

– Hello Sunday The Retouch One SPF 30

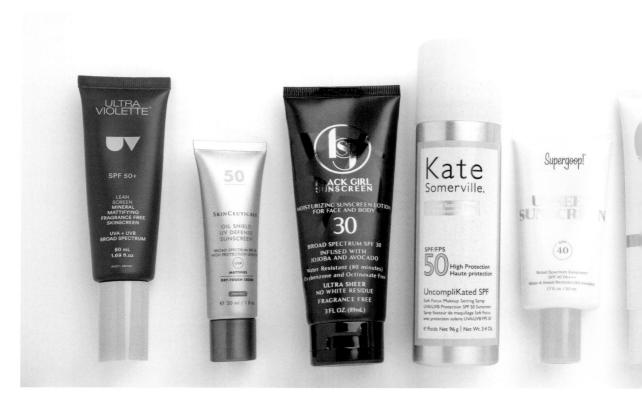

- Chemical SPFs contain chemical carbon absorbers like oxybenzone, octinoxate and avobenzone, which absorb the UV rays, convert them into heat and then release them from the body.

There are positives and negatives to using both, so this is a case of personal preference. Neither are perfect at protecting the skin from the sun. Chemical is better for those that don't like the idea of using titanium or zinc on the skin, however, the chemical carbon absorbers can cause clogging of the skin. Adapt to what suits your skin.

TIMING

When you've applied your SPF, just be sure to give it some time to sink in before you go ahead with any makeup or primers. A few minutes will do, it just means it has some time to be absorbed. It will be better for your skin and better for your makeup.

SPF FOR DRY SKIN:

- Shiseido Expert Sun Protector Face and Body Lotion SPF 50

- Bondi Sands Sunscreen Lotion SPF 50+

- La Roche-Posay Anthelios Age Correct SPF 50+

- Ultra Violette Supreme Screen Hydrating Facial Sunscreen SPF 50+

- Ultrasun Face SPF 50

- Garnier Ambre Solaire SPF 50

- Supergoop Glow Stick SPF 50

- Sarah Chapman Skinesis Skin Insurance SPF 50

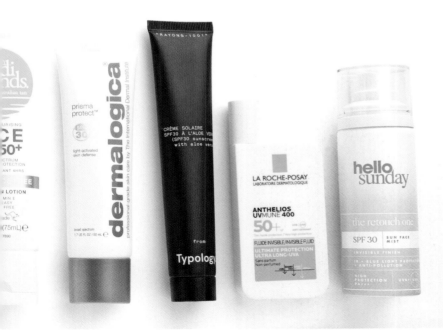

Primers

This is the point at which you may think to use a primer, but I must say I have a bit of a confession to make here . . . and that's that I don't really use primers! I know, I know, surely a makeup artist uses a makeup primer? But I rarely do.

The thing is, I want base makeup to look like skin. I want it to melt in and become a second skin. Good skincare helps facilitate this, whereas I've found some primers actually create a barrier between your skin and the makeup, preventing your makeup from sitting properly.

If my Instagram DMs are anything to go by, I think your average consumer is pretty confused by primers. It is often thought of as a hero product that will help your makeup stick like glue and perfects the look of the skin, but I have found that's so rarely the case. What's going to make your makeup look good is how well you've prepped your skin beforehand – think back to the cake analogy at the start of this chapter.

Primer:
This is a preparatory product applied to the skin aiming to create a canvas to hold whatever makeup is applied on top.

———

Silicone:
Is derived from silica and is used in beauty products to create a silky, smooth, blurred finish to the skin.

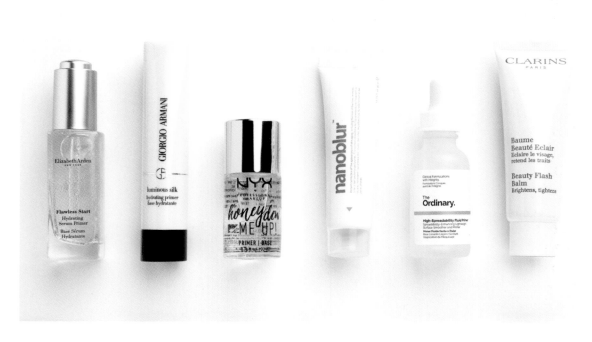

Lots of makeup primers also contain a lot of silicone, which on first application has a wonderful smoothing effect, which is why people often assume that primer is all that's necessary prior to makeup but, my goodness, you couldn't be more wrong! Silica or silicone is oil-absorbing, which is great if you're really worried about excess oil production, but if your skin is dry, it will make your skin look and feel dry and tight. It can also mean that when applied on top, foundation can look a little streaky. If this is happening to you and you're using a makeup primer, take a look at the ingredients – it's probably the silicone content.

Now, just to completely contradict myself, there are some primers that work wonderfully – bear with me! Usually, the benefit these primers bring to your skin before makeup is due to colour correction or illumination, not because they magically help your makeup to last longer.

One example that springs to mind is the desire to control redness in the skin before makeup. There are a number of green- and yellow-toned primers that, thanks to their colour, do indeed correct and tone down the red. There are also pink- and lavender-toned primers that help brighten a sallow-looking complexion, and gorgeous illuminating primers that I like to use to create that 'lit from within glow' to a makeup look, rather than using more obvious highlighters over makeup.

Colour correction and luminosity are the key benefits of primers, not magical skin perfection or makeup adhesion. I know I'm labouring the point, but that's because I'm so passionate about it!

PRIMERS I LIKE:

– Bobbi Brown Vitamin Enriched Face Base

– Clarins Beauty Flash Balm

– Armani Luminous Silk Hydrating Primer

– e.l.f. Hydrating Face Primer

PORE-MINIMISING PRIMERS:

– Benefit The POREfessional Face Primer

– Trinny London Miracle Blur

– Estée Lauder The Smoother Universal Perfecting Primer

– Smashbox Photo Finish Minimize Pores

MATTIFYING PRIMERS:

– Bobbi Brown Primer Plus Mattifier

– Shiseido Synchro Skin Soft Blurring Primer

– Paula's Choice Shine Stopper

– Hourglass Veil Mineral Primer

ILLUMINATING PRIMERS:

– Charlotte Tilbury Wonderglow

– Clarins SOS Primer Universal Light

– Laura Mercier Pure Canvas Illuminating Primer

– Beauty Pie All-In-Wonder Tinted Illuminating Primer

– Elemis Superfood Glow Priming Moisturiser

– Sculpted By Aimee Beauty Base Pearl

– VIEVE Skin Nova

– Rare Beauty Always An Optimist Illuminating Primer

– Barry M Fresh Face Illuminating Primer

– Max Factor Miracle Prep Illuminating & Hydrating Primer

– MAC Studio Radiance Primer

– Benefit That Gal Brightening Face Primer

Whilst most of what I've just said isn't ground-breaking, I do hope it has helped you understand how best to prep your skin before makeup. It is worth taking the time and making the effort to get this stage right.

> *Always be sure to have clean hands before you start your skincare routine – and to all MUAs reading this, remember: always use a tool to access your skincare if you have products in tubs – never double dip!*

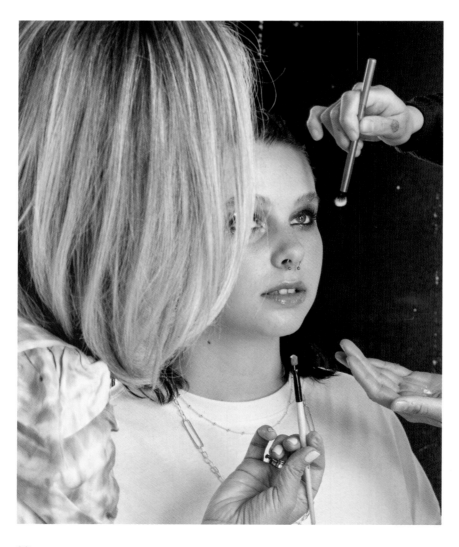

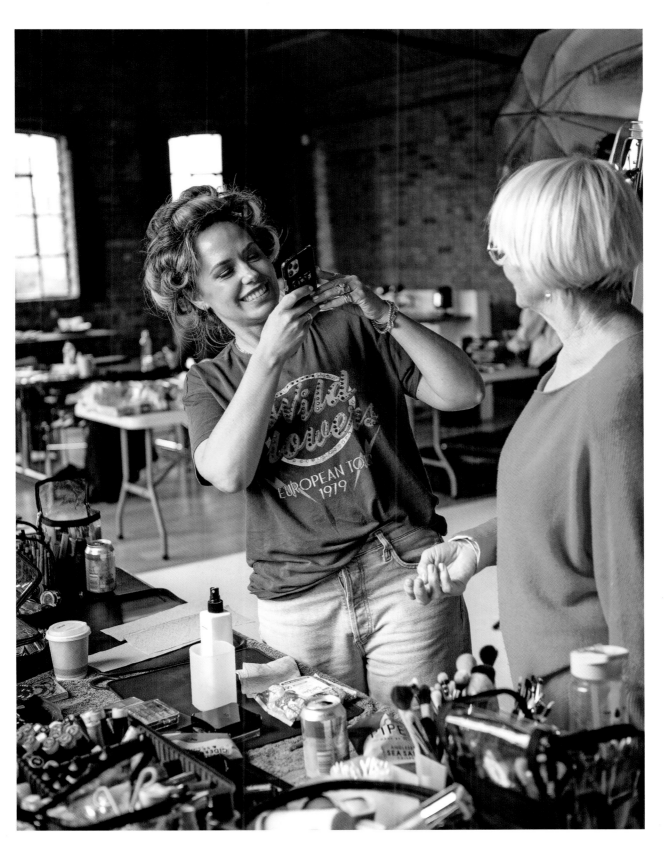

THE BASE:
FOUNDATION

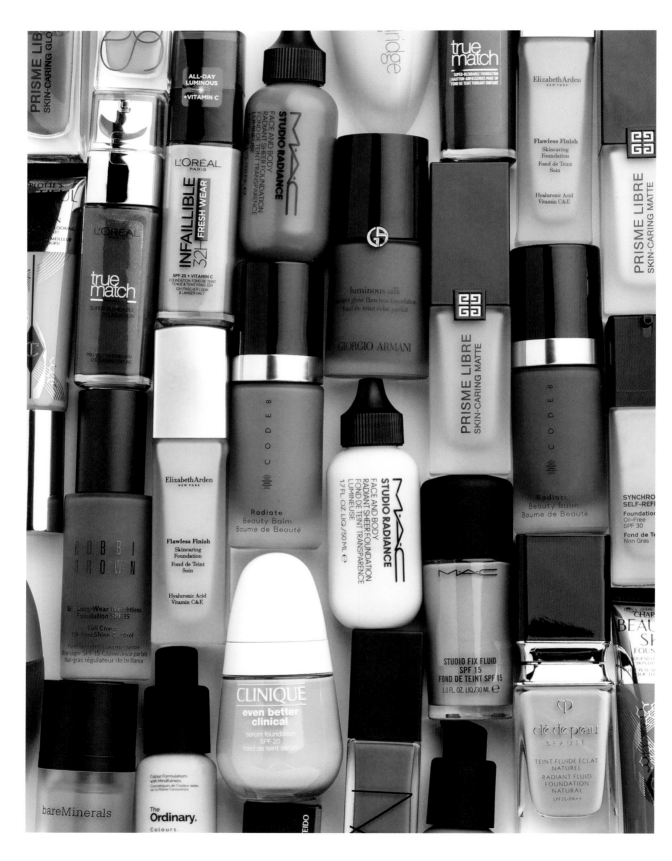

THE BASE: FOUNDATION

I do love foundation. I've just done a quick count and in the drawers next to me – don't judge me – I've found 89. Even I'm surprised I have so many. I must have a clear-out!

> *I suppose, like many of you, I am on the eternal quest for the holy grail foundation. I'm not sure I've found it yet, but I do have a number that I love and adore for different reasons.*

The thing with foundations is that they come in so many different forms, textures and finishes that there are multiple options for everyone. Which one you choose depends on your skin type but also the finish you desire, from tinted moisturisers to CC and BB creams, liquids, powders, sticks and more!

In light of this, I think it's probably best if I break down foundations by category and benefit or it could get confusing! Buying a foundation can be an overwhelming experience with so many variables affecting how it sits and looks on the skin, and I understand that for many, makeup is a non-essential luxury and buying multiple formulas simply isn't an option, so let's unpick how you can choose the right one for you.

Our skin is probably the biggest factor in guiding our foundation choice, along with preference of finish, but frustratingly our skin behaves differently from day to day, meaning a foundation that sat beautifully on your skin one day might not look so good on another.

Knowing how to identify how your skin is and knowing how to 'treat' it is the key. I'll use a classic example to explain what I mean.

Imagine you're going for a night out with your friends. You had a great sleep the night before, you'd been drinking lots of water and taking care of your skin. You exfoliated, did a hydrating sheet mask to prep, used all your favourite skincare and took your time with your makeup and getting ready.

You have a brilliant time with your friends, get home late, crawl into bed with your makeup on and catch a few hours' sleep before having to get up for work the next day. You get up in a rush, take your makeup off in the shower with your body wash (hands up anyone guilty of doing this once in a while), quickly pop on your moisturiser, followed by foundation, grab a coffee and off you go.

> *Lack of sleep, dehydration, not enough skincare, consumption of alcohol and sugar, insufficient cleansing, irritating cleanser (body wash in this case!) etc., etc., will take its toll on your skin. The foundation you wore the day before that made your skin look glorious, simply won't look the same.*

Knowing that after such a time your skin might be different will help you make better choices for it. A more hydrating serum, perhaps a richer moisturiser and, more importantly in this case, a different foundation.

I know that when my skin is tired and dehydrated, it will actually look much better not in my 'special occasion, slightly more coverage' foundation but in a lighter tinted moisturiser to which I can add concealer to perfect where needed.

Our skin usually feels different from season to season, too, with people most commonly reporting that their skin feels drier in winter, thanks to things like cold air and central heating, and oilier in summer, due to our skin naturally secreting oil as we sweat. Whilst we can manipulate foundation with skincare, I'll explain how one solution might be to use different foundation formulas that you may already have.

If you have a foundation that, for whatever reason, feels a little too dry, then in this case I'd suggest using a little more skincare before you apply it or mixing it with your moisturiser or hydrating serum. For example, **Charlotte Tilbury's Airbrush Flawless Foundation** makes for an excellent base, as a little goes a long way and it really does create a flawless finish, but you don't have a lot of time to blend as the texture is fairly 'stiff' and will dry quickly. It can drag on the skin if you haven't used enough skincare. If you naturally have drier skin, you might think you couldn't wear this texture, but if you layer your hydrating products and create a lot of slip to your skin (i.e. if you run your finger down your cheek and there's a bit of a wet look and no dryness) it will glide on easily, as it is supported by base emollients.

Alternatively, let's flip this and say you have oily skin but you want to wear the **YSL Touche Éclat foundation**, which is synonymous with glow, but worry that it will simply slide off your face. You can then use a water-based moisturiser, which won't add any unwanted oil to the skin. If you're excessively oily, you can skip moisturiser altogether, maybe just use a hydrating face mist and rely on the hydration in the makeup. Another option is to apply an oil-absorbing, mattifying primer like **Nars Pore & Shine Control Primer**, which, thanks to the silica in it, absorbs oil as it comes through the skin and stops it, or at least delays it, from coming through your makeup. Afterwards, apply the foundation but set through the T-zone or wherever you secrete more oil with an oil-free loose powder to lock it in place, leaving the other areas of the face to glow.

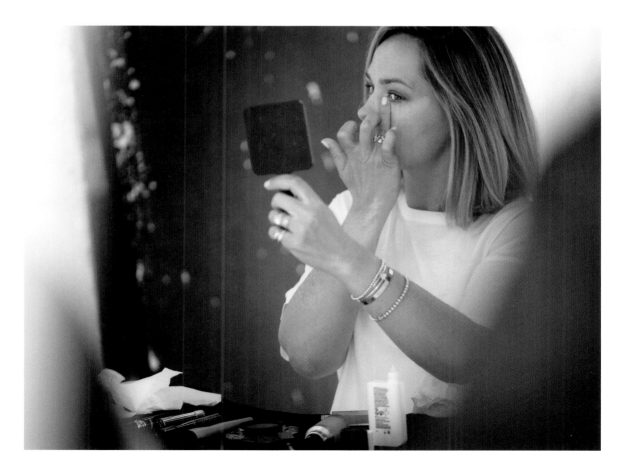

Tinted moisturiser

Tints are perfect for those days when you don't fancy wearing much makeup but want something to even out your skin tone a little and add some hydration to the skin.

A common misconception is that tinted moisturisers can replace the need for a moisturiser first, but that's not the case. It may be that because you are going to wear a tinted moisturiser you can use less of your skincare beforehand, but in my experience, even a tint sits better on already hydrated skin.

Due to tinted moisturisers being much more sheer than foundation formulas (because they contain less pigment and more moisturiser) it is much easier to choose a shade that suits you as you can see your skin through it. For example, MAC Cosmetics make 67 shades of their Studio Fix Foundation but only 30 of their Studio Radiance Face and Body, because it's a much sheerer product. When choosing your shade, if possible it's best to try it out on your face, right in the centre and across the cheek. Do not test on the neck or the back of the hand as usually they have no real comparison to the tone of your face. But if you aren't able to go to the store, then most brands have excellent virtual try-on facilities on their website. If you choose to use these functions, be sure to do so then when your skin is makeup-free and in a good light so that the technology can match to your true skin tone as best as it can.

APPLICATION

I like to apply tints with clean fingers as the warmth of my hands helps to melt the makeup into the skin. Simply dot over your forehead, cheeks, nose and chin and blend. You can of course use brushes or a sponge if you prefer, but be mindful that these (which you should always wet beforehand and then wring out the excess water) tend to absorb liquid products, so you might find you use much more than if you were to blend with your fingers.

EQUIPMENT

As I've said, I like to use clean fingers to apply moisturiser, but you can also use a synthetic brush (either a flat foundation brush or domed foundation/base brush) or a sponge.

TINTED MOISTURISERS I LIKE:

– bareMinerals Complexion Rescue

– Bobbi Brown Nude Finish Tinted Moisturiser

– Beauty Pie Super Healthy Skin Sheer Tinted Moisturiser

– Laura Mercier Tinted Moisturiser

– Nars Pure Radiant Tinted Moisturiser

– Shiseido Synchro Skin Self Refreshing Tint

– Code8 Radiate Beauty Balm

– Chantecaille Just Skin Tinted Moisturiser

– Armani Neo Nude Glow

– Morphe Glowstunner Hydrating Tinted Moisturiser

– Rose Inc Skin Enhance Luminous Tinted Serum

– Rare Beauty Positive Light Tinted Moisturiser

THE LOOK

Tinted moisturisers do vary in coverage but usually they are fairly sheer and leave the skin with a bit of a glow. For some, this is plenty of base product, while for others, this wouldn't be anywhere near enough. However, I do love a casual, pared-back base makeup look sometimes, and a tint is a great way to achieve this.

WHO IS IT BEST FOR?

Tints aren't just for those that want a glow or have dry or dehydrated skin. There are plenty of oil-free versions available that are suitable for more oily-skin types. I should say, though, that because of their very nature, tinted moisturisers aren't the most long-wearing of bases and they can be prone to sliding in the heat, so be mindful of this.

This may be surprising to some, but I actually love to use oil-free tinted moisturisers on acneic skin. It just works to start with a light layer of base and then use concealer to conceal redness.

> *Sometimes, too heavy or dry a foundation over blemishes can actually highlight their texture and be less flattering. Using a tinted moisturiser also means you don't have to apply heavy foundation to the clearer areas of skin.*

*

Acneic skin:
Skin that is prone to acne. Acne is most common in oily skin but can occur in those with dry skin too. Acne occurs when hair follicles become blocked with oil and dead skin cells causing whiteheads, blackheads and spots.

MAKE YOUR OWN TINTED MOISTURISER

If you don't have a tinted moisturiser but like the idea of something a little more lightweight, you can always add some of your current foundation to a moisturiser, mix in the palm of your hand and try that to see how the more sheer coverage looks.

BB and CC creams

These fit into the tinted moisturiser family, but as the categories have expanded and gained popularity, I think some are confused regarding the difference between the formulations. BB cream was first created by a German dermatologist (Dr Christine Schrammek) back in the sixties to help protect her patients' skin after they'd had laser and chemical peel treatments, which can leave skin incredibly vulnerable. She called the product Blemish Balm and it contained high SPF, skincare and pigment. As word spread about her Blemish Balm, cosmetics companies followed suit and made their own.

Possibly some of the key attributes got lost over time and maybe they aren't all as powerful as the original, but I'd say now that a classic BB cream is similar to a tinted moisturiser but with a much higher SPF – usually 40 or more. Rather than being known as 'Blemish Balm', here in the UK they are now more commonly called Beauty Balms, which is somewhat more palatable. However, essentially what used to be fairly specialised is now usually more of a classic tinted moisturiser.

The 'CC' in CC cream stands for 'colour correction' and because of that, they come in many shades and guises. Some CC creams have gone down

BB & CC CREAMS I LIKE:

– Erborian BB Cream

– Erborian Super BB – if you like a bit more coverage

– Trinny London BFF

– IT Cosmetics Your Skin But Better CC+ Cream

– Erborian CC Cream

– Clinique Moisture Surge CC Cream

– Olay Total Effects CC Cream

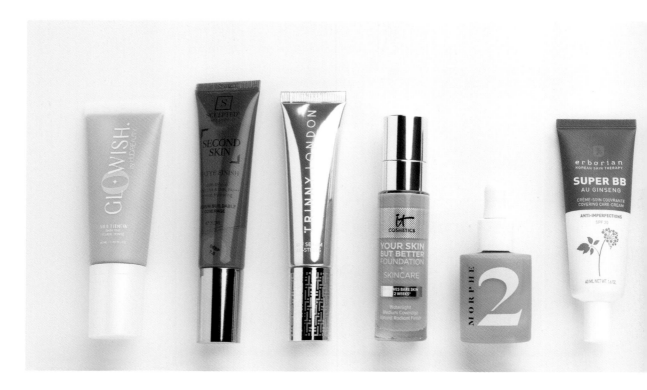

the physically coloured route to create different shades, usually pastels, to help correct unwanted colour in the skin. If you look at a traditional colour wheel, it's the colours opposite each other that cancel each other out. Traditionally, green and yellow CC creams help control redness, lilac neutralises yellow, pinky tones can brighten dullness and oranges are great for neutralising dark shadows and pigmentation.

However, similar to BB creams, it seems that CC creams now come in many shades that mirror natural skin tones, and they act more like a tinted moisturiser or foundation would, however, the onus is still on their ability to neutralise and colour correct the skin.

APPLICATION

Same as for tinted moisturisers, see page 46.

EQUIPMENT

Clean fingers or a synthetic brush. Use either a flat foundation brush or domed foundation/base brush. You can also use a sponge.

Pigmentation:
This means colouring. The pigment in our skin is called melanin and is produced by the melanocyte cells in the basal layer of the epidermis. Skin pigmentation disorders affect the colour of your skin. Hyper-pigmentation causes your skin to darken in areas and vitiligo causes areas of light skin.

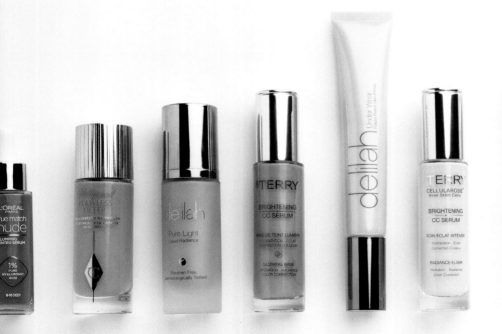
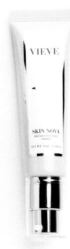

Testing Foundations

Testing foundation is key. When looking for a new foundation, the first step is to pick a colour match that you are happy with. You then have two options – either take a sample home and try it with your preferred skincare and see how it wears for a day or two, or remove your base makeup completely/go in with a clean face and apply a full face of the foundation in the store (each store will have differing post Covid protocols for this, but most brands will offer foundation matching services) and see how it wears.

Do not try the makeup on the back of your hand. It is a complete waste of time and won't help you make a good decision. Your hands are not only a different shade than your face (in most cases), but the skin is also a totally different texture. The only way to know how a foundation wears and feels is by applying it as you would normally.

I emphasise this as I've spent my career trying to help people find the right base makeup and all too often when the texture or colour isn't right, the client has either been shown it on the back of their hands, on their neck (usually significantly paler than the face), on the chest (often significantly warmer than the face) or on the jawline in too small a patch to really be able to tell.

When it comes to finding the right shade, you want to make sure that as you apply the foundation to the skin, preferably clean skin in the centre of the face, the shade almost disappears – this obviously indicates that it's a good match.

The key here is that you shouldn't need to 'blend' too much. Just tap the edge of the makeup as, realistically, most shades that are near to your skin tone will look ok if they are blended really well but they may look wrong if applied all over.

If you're happy with the foundation shade on the cheek, then do always also check it on the forehead as this part of the face is usually a touch warmer. If the pigment is significantly warmer there, I often end up having to use two foundations to get the best match. You may need a deeper shade around the corners of the face and a lighter one through the centre. Yes, it might be annoying having two foundations on the go at the same time, but they will last longer as you're using just a little of each at a time.

*

Full coverage: This type of foundation is designed to cover the skin completely, but you can of course customise a full coverage foundation by sheering it out with a moisturiser.

In fact, it is rare for your skin to be the same tone all over, as most of us have areas of hyperpigmentation. It is particularly common in those with black and brown skin that has more melanin present. If the melanocytes are damaged by the sun or other factors, then they will produce extra melanin, resulting in areas of darker skin otherwise known as hyperpigmentation. The best thing to prevent this condition is the daily use of SPF but there are lots of skincare products available to help treat and minimise areas of discolouration. Vitamin C has long been spoken of as an ingredient to help with pigmentation, but aesthetician and black skin expert Dija Ayodele recommends the use of specialised fading serums like **Cosmedix Simply Brilliant 24/7 Brightening Serum** and **Skinbetter Science Even Tone Correcting Serum**. I would highly recommend reading her book *Black Skin* for more information on this. To correct or even out areas of hyperpigmentation using makeup, it can be helpful to use a peach- or yellow-coloured corrector under your foundation. The corrector neutralises and brightens the areas of discolouration so your foundation looks even on top.

> *If the foundation is really obvious on the skin, either lighter or deeper than your skin tone, then it's not right.*

The above seems almost ridiculous to write this, as it's not rocket science and to many it's common knowledge, but there are so many people that struggle to find the right shade of foundation that I'm including some advice here. If your take-away from this section is just that going forward you'll test a foundation before you buy, and that you'll test the shade through the centre of the face, then it's been worth writing!

Please don't be afraid to ask for help. In department stores, the makeup artists on the counters have been trained in the products they're selling and can guide you to the right choice, both in formula and shade. However, you should never let a makeup artist convince you of a shade. If you're not sure, listen to your gut, as it's usually right. If in doubt do ask to stand in natural light to take a better look and be sure to look into a mirror straight on. I often see people checking foundation shades looking down whilst holding a hand-held mirror – usually causing shadows to fall across the face and making it hard to see the shade accurately. Instead, hold the mirror slightly above your eyeline so that you are looking up, with your face catching more light. This will allow you to see the true colour of the foundation on your skin.

Stick foundation

When talking about stick foundation, I know lots of people panic, assuming that all products are like the Pan Stik, developed and made famous by Max Factor, the legendary Hollywood film makeup artist back in the 1940s. Thick and heavy, it was designed to make actors' skin look even in a new era of cinematography and bright lights.

There has been a lot of development in cosmetics since then, and now there are lots of different textures of stick foundation available to suit all skin types and with a number of finishes. From matte, long-wearing formulas to lightweight moisturising ones, actually some of my favourite foundations come in stick form!

APPLICATION

The joy of a stick foundation is that you can completely control the coverage you achieve. For light coverage, use your fingers to dab stick foundation just in the areas that you want to even out. For medium coverage, use a foundation brush with a stick foundation to buff into the skin. For full coverage, swipe the stick directly onto the skin and blend either with fingers, a brush or a makeup sponge.

EQUIPMENT

Clean fingers, a brush or a sponge.

THE LOOK

A foundation stick allows you to customise your look. For example, you could use minimal skincare, apply a lot of the stick and you're left with a matte, full-coverage base. Alternatively, apply less to well-hydrated skin for a more lightweight application or use the tiniest bit for more of a tinted moisturiser feel ... it's up to you. A foundation stick is incredibly flexible, which is why I am such a fan and really encourage you to give one a go!

WHO IS IT BEST FOR?

Above all, stick foundations are so handy! Slim and portable, they can go in your handbag as a convenient touch-up item. Cream foundations in pots are much like sticks, just packaged differently. Makeup artists Keyvn Aucoin and, more recently, Monika Blunder, have released versions.

STICK FOUNDATION I LIKE:

– Bobbi Brown Skin Foundation Stick

– bareMinerals Complexion Rescue Hydrating Foundation Stick

– Huda Beauty Fauxfilter Skin Finish

– Hourglass Vanish Seamless Finish Foundation Stick

– Tom Ford Traceless Foundation Stick

– Revolution Fast Base Foundation Stick

– Lancôme Teint Idole Foundation Stick

– Kiko Active Foundation Long Lasting Stick Foundation

– MAC Studio Fix Soft Matte Foundation Stick

Powder foundation

While I personally prefer to use liquid foundations, there is absolutely a place for powder foundation in my makeup collection.

APPLICATION

For many, a powdered foundation is a comfort zone they don't ever wish to leave! Often it's because it's the first texture they were introduced to when experimenting with makeup and convenience is a huge benefit. Simply sweep the powder over the skin with the sponge it comes with (just be sure to wash it regularly) or use a brush to apply for lighter coverage. There's none of the mess, or risk of mess, you can have with a liquid, unless you smash it, open the case and have the powder crumble all over the floor – and I can safely say that we've all been there!

EQUIPMENT

For lighter coverage, apply with a powder brush. For more full coverage apply with a sponge or makeup pad.

WHO IS IT BEST FOR?

For lots of people with oily skin, there's an assumption that a powder will be better for them and more mattifying. Whilst that's often the case, it's not always true because many powder foundations also contain oil and can add moisture to the skin – which is no bad thing, of course, just not what people have been led to believe. The danger is that a powder foundation can make the skin look dull and flat, but prep your skin following my skincare advice and that simply won't be the case.

THE LOOK

The reason I own a few powdered foundations, despite being a fan of a more dewy look, is because sometimes powder can disguise texture. I don't mean scabs or flakes, as powder will, of course, exacerbate their appearance. I'm talking about really delicate, wafer-thin skin that when you apply liquid foundation looks awful. Does this sound familiar? It's something I've encountered a lot more in recent years thanks to the rise in popularity and availability of acids and retinoids. Lots of people I've worked with, myself included, have arrived on set having gone to town the night before with their retinol in the hope of waking up to gloriously clear, exfoliated skin, but have in fact burnt their skin and not allowed enough time for the skin to repair.

How this translates on the skin is as teeny-tiny flakes, not necessarily visible to the naked eye during skin prep but which become really obvious when you try to apply liquid foundation. It's as if minute pigment particles manage to get themselves tucked into all the tiny creases and no amount of blending or skin prep can fix it – I should know, I've tried! You can't correct the issue with skincare and face oil, you will need to cleanse, reapply skincare and then use a powder foundation. It will work like magic!

MINERAL MAKEUP

I'll touch on mineral makeup here as, although not exclusively, many come in powder form. Formulated with ground minerals and fewer of the additives you find in liquid foundations, mineral makeup is often marketed as good for sensitive skin because the ingredients are all natural.

Mineral makeup is also often recommended for those with acneic skin as it's classed as non-comedogenic, meaning it doesn't clog pores and cause blemishes, instead it sits on top of and smooths over pores.

POWDER FOUNDATION I LIKE:

– MAC Studio Fix Powder

– L'Oréal Infallible 24hr Fresh Wear Powder Foundation

– Shiseido Synchro Skin Invisible Loose Powder

– Chantecaille Compact Makeup Foundation

– bareMinerals Barepro Pressed 16hr Foundation

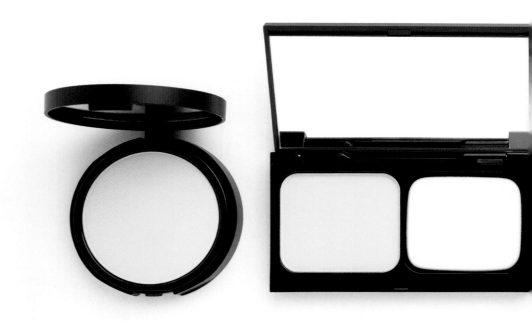

Mineral makeup also creates a physical barrier to the sun, as most contain the minerals zinc oxide and titanium dioxide. However, it's actually because of this that I don't use mineral makeup on the red carpet or on my brides, instead sticking to SPF under liquid foundation, because it's these minerals that can cause flashback in flash photography. This means that the foundation, which was a perfect colour match in natural daylight, suddenly has a very pale, whitish glow when it bounces the light of the flash. Definitely not what we are aiming for!

I learnt this the hard way during a photoshoot in my very short-lived modelling days as a teenager. I'd worn what looked like a great foundation but it was SPF 30, and when the photographer developed the photos, I looked like I had a very bizarre floating white head (and yes, I'll see if I can find the evidence and share it with you all!).

Minerals also attract oil, so whilst you might think you'd rather use a mineral powder foundation because you have oily skin, mineral makeup can grow increasingly more 'wet' as your skin produces sebum. I do like to use mineral makeup on occasion, but these are just things to be wary of to meet your skin's differing needs.

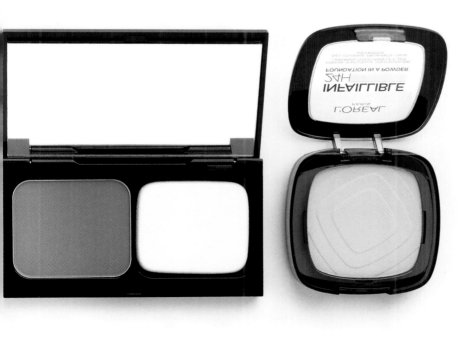

Liquid foundation

I expect most of us that are interested in makeup or like to wear makeup will own or will have owned a liquid foundation. However, of all the makeup categories, this is the one that varies the most. There are literally hundreds, if not thousands, of different textures and finishes, not to mention different colours.

Essentially, there's every finish imaginable available for liquid foundations, from really light, barely-there formulas to slightly more pigmented ones that offer medium coverage and thicker, full-coverage ones, all of which can be hydrating and glowy or oil-free and matte.

Choosing which one is right for you essentially comes down to your skin type and your preference to finish.

WHICH FINISH?

Those with **dry/dehydrated** skin will probably best suit a **more hydrating finish**, which will add moisture and oil to the skin so it looks plump and balanced and the makeup flatters the skin.

Those with **oily skin** might better suit an **oil-free one**, which won't add unwanted or excess oil to the skin so the base adheres, looks semi-matte and less shiny – the coverage level is simply a matter of preference.

However, the obvious caveat here is that, of course, a dry/dehydrated skin can wear an oil-free foundation. I simply hope to explain that if you buy an oil-free, long-wearing base and have dry or dehydrated skin, you might not love how it looks and feels. Alternatively, if your skin is on the oily side and you purchase a rich, hydrating formula, you might find it comes off easily.

*

Hydrated:
Hydrated skin has a good balance of water and oil in its surface layer and presents as healthy looking, smooth and often with a seemingly natural glow.

Dehydrated:
Dehydrated skin has a lack of water and oil in the surface layer of the skin and can present as flaky, dull and dry.

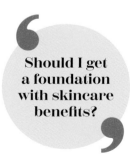

Should I get a foundation with skincare benefits?

Ingredients in liquid foundations vary hugely too. Many foundations focus just on makeup and coverage, but lots of brands have seen an opportunity to add skincare to their bases, tapping into the consumers who want to take care of their skin whilst also making it look good. My take here is that skincare shouldn't be omitted or replaced by a, let's say, serum-infused foundation. Also, the addition of skincare ingredients will impact the price point, so whilst some formulas are indeed worthy of their price and contain skin-loving ingredients, my personal preference is to buy skincare for its ingredients and benefits and then makeup for its finish and wear, not its skincare claims. Anyone else's mind go immediately to the 'honey and apricot' scene in *Notting Hill*?

SAMPLES

Ask to take a foundation sample home so you can see for yourself. Brands want your custom, so most will be more than happy to oblige if they can. However, I will share from years of experience in retail that sample pots are like gold dust. In one store I worked in, I had to hide my sample pots as they would otherwise go missing and they were essential to my business. So, if a makeup artist tells you they don't have a sample pot, then they're most likely telling the truth.

I therefore suggest that if you know you're going to go foundation shopping, take some kind of pot with you so that you have something you can take a sample away in. All you need is five pumps of foundation, which equates to a few days' worth. It doesn't look like much, but trust me it's enough to see if you like the product. You don't need to fill a 10ml pot, and makeup artists can't give away that much of a sample anyway.

The bottom line, though, is please never buy a foundation out of obligation or if you're unsure. The chances are you'll have wasted your money.

FINISH

Liquid foundations vary hugely in finish due to their formula. So whilst there are formulas that are more suitable for different skin types, you can also choose your foundation based on the finish you desire.

A basic rule of thumb is:

· Those with **dry skin** will benefit from **hydrating formulas**, which have an onus on illumination and glow.

· Those with more **oily skin** might be better suited to **oil-free formulas**.

However, neither is off-limits for either skin type. A dry skin type can wear oil-free makeup and vice versa. You will simply need to use skincare to prep the skin appropriately. For example, **if you have dry skin but like the look of a more matte, full-coverage, oil-free makeup**, you'll need to ensure you have prepped the skin well beforehand or it could make your skin look flat and dull.

HYDRATING FOUNDATION I LIKE:

– Urban Decay Hydromaniac

– L'Oréal True Match Nude

– MAC Studio Radiance Face and Body

– YSL Touche Éclat Le Teint Foundation

– Shiseido Synchro Skin Radiant

– Armani Luminous Silk

– Clé de Peau Beauté Radiant Fluid Foundation

– Kevyn Aucoin Etherealist Illuminating Foundation

– Charlotte Tilbury Beautiful Skin

– Nars Sheer Glow

– IT Cosmetics Your Skin But Better

– Sisley Phyto Teint Nude

– Illamasqua Beyond Foundation

– Nars Light Reflecting Foundation

– Urban Decay Stay Naked

– Chanel Les Beiges

So, a little scrub with an exfoliating facewash is a great place to start to help lift off any dead, dry skin cells, then follow with my recommended routine of essence, eye cream, serum, moisturiser and SPF (see pages 20–39), but you may want to layer a light oil under your SPF to ensure the skin is as hydrated and supple as possible before you apply the more matte foundation.

Alternatively, **if you have oily skin but want a glow from your base**, then by all means use a hydrating base but maybe scale back the skincare so you don't overload the skin with emollients.

Stick to essence after cleansing and eye cream, but use your lightest water-based gel cream in order to keep the oil in your skincare to a minimum. On some rare occasions, those with extremely oily skin might skip moisturiser altogether and rely on the hydrating benefits of the essence and foundation combined. Depending on how oily the skin is, you might prefer to omit moisturiser altogether. I know that sounds sacrilege for us skincare obsessives but you may find there's enough moisture in the hydrating base that your skin simply doesn't need anymore and the essence will be all that's needed to balance the skin. However, don't confuse this with me having previously said that those with oily skin must use moisturiser. I stand by that – oily skin can still become dehydrated as previously explained – my advice here is simply for those moments when you wish to manipulate your usual makeup prep to enable you to use a foundation which conventionally may not suit your skin type.

Cushion compact foundations

Cushion compacts first appeared in Korea, from where the 'K-beauty' trend spread globally, and were designed as handy high-SPF foundations that you can apply on the go – a way of topping up your sun protection without ruining your makeup. In most cases, a cushion compact is a circular compact just a bit chunkier than a powder one, which contains a sponge soaked in foundation at the bottom and a second tier containing a sponge applicator. The idea is that you press the soaked sponger with your applicator sponge and press gently over the face. Coverage tends to be medium, often with a dewy finish and with an emphasis on sun protection and skincare. They're not hugely popular in the UK, but they are available and are an excellent option for those that take their sun care seriously.

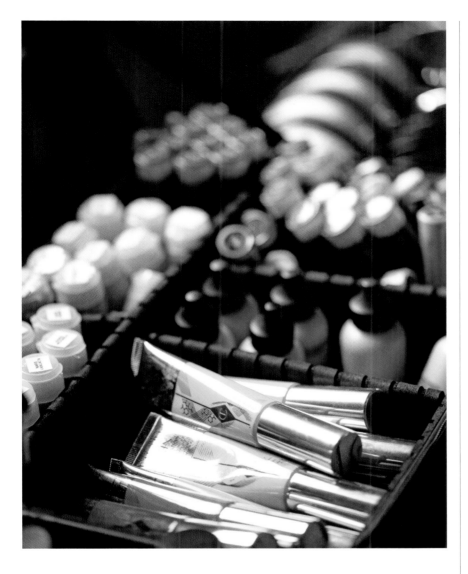

LONG-WEAR FOUNDATION I LIKE:

- Estée Lauder Double Wear
- L'Oréal True Match
- Fenty Pro Filt'r Foundation
- MAC Studio Fix
- MAC Pro Longwear
- Sculpted By Aimee Satin Silk
- Delilah Alibi The Perfect Cover
- Charlotte Tilbury Airbrush Flawless Foundation
- Lisa Eldridge The Foundation
- Max Factor Facefinity
- Lancôme Teint Idole
- Laura Mercier Flawless Fusion Ultra-Longwear
- L'Oréal Infallible 24hr Fresh Wear Foundation
- Clé de Peau Beauté Radiant Fluid
- Hourglass Vanish Seamless Finish Foundation
- bareMinerals Barepro
- Huda Beauty Fauxfilter Luminous Matte

I learnt this fact at a press junket I was doing for an actress who had really oily skin. She told me not to use moisturiser, which I couldn't believe and was reluctant to proceed without, but she was absolutely right. She had very active sebaceous glands and didn't need a moisturiser under makeup. If I had applied moisturiser, then her makeup would have simply slid off, and that's the last thing you need when you have a day of back-to-back interviews followed by a red carpet appearance for your film premiere! Essence can be enough and sometimes an oil-controlling lotion can be helpful throughout the T-zone to absorb some of the oil before it comes through the makeup.

Undertones

I have found throughout my career that many struggle to identify the undertone of their skin. It can be overwhelming and it is easy to be confused by the brands that market their foundation by undertone.

The three undertones are cool, warm and neutral. Those with cool tones will see blues and pinks in their skin. Those with warm skin tones see mainly golden tints, such as yellow and peach, and those with neutral undertones won't see extremes of either pink or gold but may see little hints of both.

There are a few easy ways to determine your skin tone. Jewellery metal preference is one of the clearest methods. If you suit silver jewellery more than anything else then you are most likely a cool undertone. If you suit gold then you're probably warm, and if you look good with mixed metals

---

HOW TO DEAL WITH PIGMENTATION

If hyperpigmentation is a concern, then you can use correctors (see page 51) to help neutralise the tone before foundation. Some dark pigmentation can make foundation applied on top look ashy, while the same shade looks great in areas not affected by the pigmentation.

To correct this, if the pigmentation is brown in tone, you can apply a peach-coloured corrector on top. It might look odd on its own, but it lifts the shadow shade and when the foundation is then applied, it prevents the shadow of the pigmentation obscuring the finish and tone of the foundation.

The deeper the pigmentation, the more intense peach you want the corrector to be. For under the eyes, it is usually a brown tone which peach will correct. Excess melanin can be produced anywhere on the face. It happens when the sun's rays damage the skin, namely the melanocytes that produce melanin. Once they're damaged, they can produce too much melanin and that's when excess pigmentation occurs. It's also common for those with black or brown skin to have naturally darker pigmentation around the mouth and under the eyes, so this would be a key area you might use a corrector on before foundation.

then you're likely a neutral. Another test to do is to look under your wrists – what colour are your veins? If they are pinky/blue then you are cool, if they're more green then you are warm and if you see both pinky/blue and green then you are neutral in tone.

Once you've identified your skin tone this will help when chosing your foundation shade. If the undertone is wrong in your foundation, it simply won't look right on your skin. If a foundation looks too pink then it's possibly too cool. If your foundation looks too yellow or orange it could be too warm. If foundation looks grey on you then it is too neutral. However, although this is helpful to know, don't let these rules overwhelm your makeup choices – you can wear whatever is your preference!

Coverage

Choosing foundation coverage is predominantly a matter of personal preference. I like to have different formulas with differing levels of coverage to suit my mood. More often than not I like the look of a lighter-weight base – I think skin looks altogether healthier with a more sheer finish and a bit of a glow – but I also love full coverge foundation on occasion, especially when going out.

What I see most commonly is people thinking they need more coverage than they actually do. Often, when you assess the concern that people want to cover it is much less significant than they think. A classic example is those with redness in the skin tone. People reach for full coverage foundation when actually the redness is often localised to around the nose or on the cheek. In these cases I suggest a foundation with lighter coverage for all over, and then just a little concealer over the area of redness. This will tone down any redness and will ensure that you are not camouflaging good-looking skin unnecessarily.

However, I understand that those with acneic skin may feel more comfortable in full coverage makeup that will completely conceal any blemishes and redness. But if your blemishes are in just one area, like around the mouth and jawline, for example, then a bit of full coverage concealer in those areas is sufficient over a lighter foundation. Most foundations are, but if acneic skin is a worry make sure to look for the term 'non-comedogenic', as this means the product has been specifically formulated so it doesn't clog pores. When pores get blocked it can lead to spots developing. If you do have blemish-prone skin then do look to use products with salycilic acid: **Sally Cleanse by Skingredients** and **Paula's Choice Skin Perfecting 2% BHA Liquid Exfoliant** are cult heroes!

Equipment

There are so many ways to apply foundation, none are 'correct' or 'right', as long as the end result is beautifully blended makeup. I'm a huge believer in whatever works best for you, but let me explain how I think the way you apply your liquid foundation affects the finish.

I have always loved using my **fingers** to apply my own base. The warmth of your fingers helps to melt the product into the skin, which I believe creates a really lightweight finish. If a client has amazing skin then I might use my fingers to apply just a little foundation around the nose, chin and cheeks – anywhere that may be a bit red or needs some colour correction. They are also the best tool for the days when you don't feel like wearing much makeup but you want your skin tone to appear even. Dab a little foundation through the centre of your face, over the nose and cheeks and a little on the chin. This creates a very pared-back, minimal makeup look.

> *I also use my fingers to apply my foundation when I am in a tearing hurry.*

Whilst I don't champion this as the optimum way of applying, I like to massage a pump of foundation between my fingertips and blend it over the face much like I would moisturiser. Note that this does not create the very best finish but it does the job!

- **A very lightly bound, fluffy brush** will create very light coverage as the soft bristles will gently move makeup where you want it. It can be tricky to blend full coverage foundations with light fluffy brushes as the hairs will struggle to move the more viscose texture across the skin, so these types of brushes are best used with tinted mositurisers and very light water-based foundations.

- **A firmer brush**, like the traditional flat foundation brush, or my Base brush from my collaboration with Ciaté London, can be beneficial when wanting a more 'made up' look as the synthetic fibres help to distribute foundation evenly across the face. When using a flat foundation brush I generally start blending foundation from the centre of the face (so from the nose) out across the cheek towards the ears. You can use as much or as little product as you like, the brush will really help distribute the foundation evenly over the skin and allow you to build the coverage to your taste. You can either brush a little all over for a more sheer finish or keep layering for full coverage.

- **A tighter-bound, flat, round-headed brush** will help create fuller coverage still as the density of the brush helps to work product into the skin. These brushes work best with full coverage foundations and don't work very well with lighter textures like tinted moisturisers, as the brustles are bound much tighter and will simply brush off the base product even if you are very light-handed when using it.

> *This theory is the same across most makeup application: the firmer the tool, the sharper, more defined the finish. The softer and fluffier the tool, the more diffused the finish will be.*

- **Sponges** are incredibly popular tools at the moment, mainly because of their prominence in social media tutorials (think YouTube, Instagram and TikTok) and their relative ease of use. Simply bounce the sponge over your face with light, repetitive dabs until all your product is evenly distributed. I don't often use them, and almost never on clients, as I'm not entirely convinced they're as hygienic to use multiple times and they're an expensive one-time purchase. I also learnt makeup application without the use of big makeup sponges, just little ones to help perfect something, such as to help blend under-eye concealer on more mature skins, a sponge lifts off less product and can dab between fine lines.

To use on yourself, the key is to soak the makeup sponge first so it fully absorbs water (the sponge will double in size!), then wring thoroughly to remove the water before use. This will ensure the sponge is nice and supple and won't absorb the foundation.

Some like to apply foundation to the sponge, then bounce over the face (and by 'bounce' I mean repeatedly tap), others prefer to dot the foundation over the face, then use the sponge to 'bounce and blend' it in.

If I use a sponge, I prefer to bounce the sponge over a finished base makeup to further blend it out, remove any possible brush marks (although clean brushes shouldn't leave any brush marks) and lift off excess product. It can be this lovely finishing touch that ensures a makeup look is a little less 'makeuppy'.

I actually prefer to use my hands to do this technique – pressing and cupping them over my client's face to help melt the makeup into the skin, then lifting off any excess product with my hands. However, I know for some this may not be possible if they have naturally oily hands, in which case you wouldn't want to transfer oil to the makeup. In this case, either a sponge or a clean foundation brush would be best.

Another technique is to spray a sponge with a face mist or hydrating setting spray and then bounce this over the skin. This will lift off any excess makeup and add a bit of moisture to the surface of the makeup, creating a softer, lighter look. An excellent hack if you feel your base is looking a bit over done and heavy.

Sponges can be really useful when someone has texture on the skin. If too much makeup is applied and the appearance of texture has been exacerbated you can 'fix' the textured look by applying a tiny bit of moisturiser to a sponge and gently tapping the area of concern. The emollients in the cream will loosen the makeup just enough to ease that caked-on look. You need to be cautious, though, as the moisturiser can lift off too much product – it's a case of using a tiny amount at a time and going bit by bit. So, this all goes to show that maybe I use sponges more than I thought and they can actually be very useful!

SPONGE HYGIENE

When it comes to sponges, hygiene is absolutely key. I've already mentioned that I don't think you can repeat-use sponges on clients but personal sponges should be cleaned after each use. If not, they can become a breeding ground for bacteria, which in turn can cause breakouts on the skin if used when dirty. A quick rinse under warm water with some mild shampoo will be sufficient, but there are lots of sponge soaps available too.

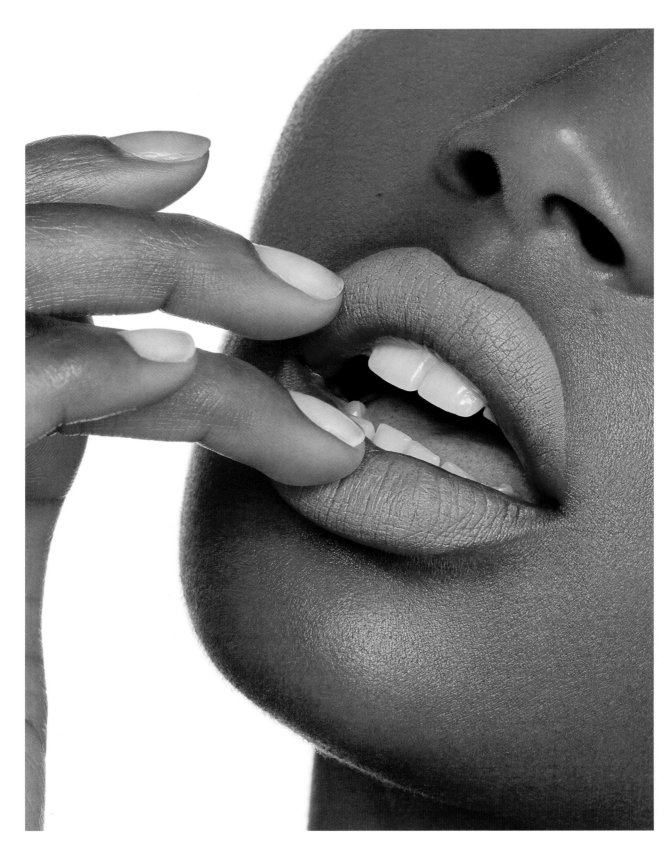

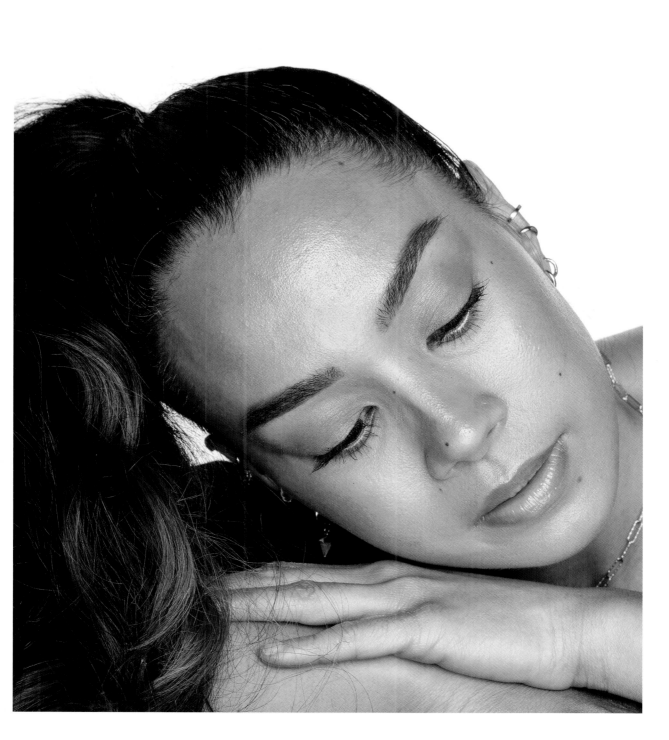

THE BASE: CONCEALER

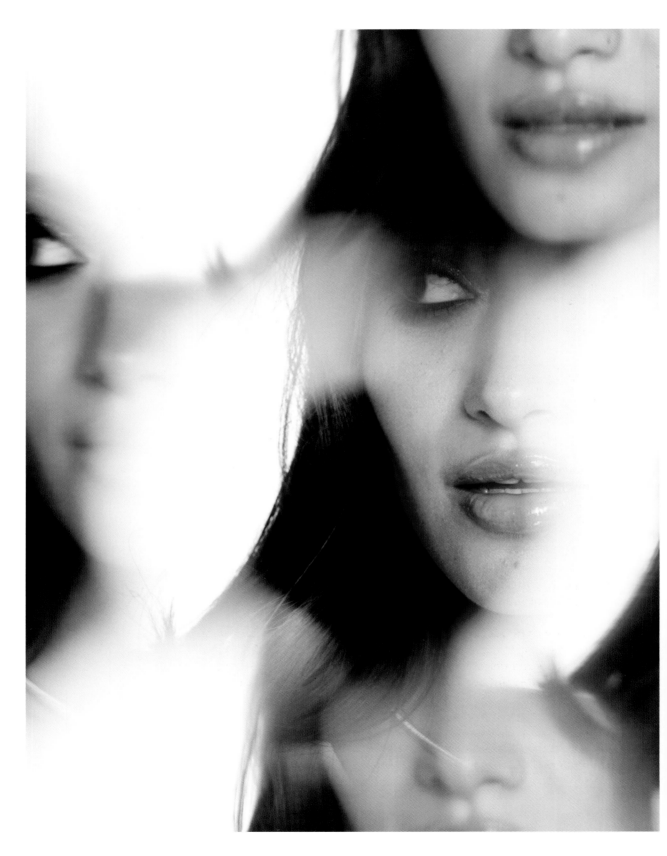

THE BASE: CONCEALER

> *When I was younger, I always assumed concealer was just for blemishes, but for the last two decades it has become one of the most important items in my makeup bag.*

This is not because I have lots of blemishes I need to hide, but because I naturally have dark under eyes and, my goodness, great under-eye concealer is a total game changer. It is often the element of my makeup that has the most transformative effect.

> *I think lots of us assume that our foundation will do the job of brightening our under eyes sufficiently, but actually a concealer can be far more effective.*

Often, foundations don't offer quite enough coverage or, if they do, the texture is so dry that it can leave the delicate skin under the eye, which is significantly thinner than anywhere else on the rest of the face, looking dry and cakey, highlighting any fine lines.

In light of this, I recommend a specific under eye concealer that is designed to better suit the skin. Of course, much like foundation, under eye concealers vary hugely in texture and finish, from super-light to full coverage. What you choose depends on a few factors:

· **If under-eye darkness isn't really a concern** for you but you want to wear a little something to even out the skin, then there's no need for anything with full coverage, unless you like that aesthetic, of course. Something very light like **RMS UnCoverup** will help create a smooth, even finish.

· **If, like me, your under eyes feel dark**, then you can opt for something altogether much thicker, like **L'Oréal Infallible** concealer. However, if you've ever tried concealer but can still see a dullness or a hint of shade poking through, then you're not alone. Lots of us experience the same thing. In this situation you might benefit from using a corrector first.

Correctors

Correctors for under the eye commonly come in two tones – pink and peach – and are used in conjunction with concealers to create a perfectly even under eye. They work by neutralising the unwanted tone first, so that when you apply your concealer on top, it's layered over a tone already significantly brighter.

Across all skin tones, pinky-toned correctors brilliantly neutralise purple and pink shadows under the eye and peach ones help neutralise brownish hues.

The intensity of the shade that you need depends on your skin tone and the depth of the shadow you wish to hide. The darker the shadow, the stronger the colour needed to counteract it. If you go too light, you could create an ashy finish to the skin.

I know some people worry about using two products under the eye and would prefer the convenience of just one, but in this case it's colour correction and layering that are key to the finish of the concealer. It's much like shampoo and conditioner: two products you use, one after the other and both different, but achieve a brilliant result when used together. Or if you imagine a freshly plastered wall, if you do just one layer of topcoat you'll most likely still see shadows and unevenness, hence the use of a base coat first.

CORRECTORS I LIKE:

- Bobbi Brown Correctors

- Charlotte Tilbury Magic Vanish

- Nars Radiant Creamy Colour Corrector

- NYX Colour Correcting Palettes

- Beauty Pie Superluminous Undereye Genius

APPLICATION

More than the dislike of using two different products, it's more common that people are concerned about how too much product under the eye will look.

If you apply a bit of eye cream before you put on your concealer, about the size of a grain of rice, the product will sit really beautifully on the skin. You want to focus your corrector **only** where you see the shadow – for most that's in the inner corner of the eye. If there's not shadow in the outer corner of your eye, then don't apply product there unnecessarily. Don't forget either side of the bridge of the nose. I specifically try to avoid placing products over the outer third of my eye, especially where it meets the top of my cheeks, as that is where I have the most fine lines. Sometimes I'll have a bit of makeup there, but it is important to keep it light.

EQUIPMENT

You can use your fingers or a brush to apply your corrector, but I always teach people to press the product into the skin using the pad of your ring finger. I see a lot of people trying to sweep or tap their correctors, but I prefer the pressing technique as I find it really works the product into the skin and removes any excess makeup at the same time, The more you work the corrector into the skin, the less obvious it's going to be. It takes a few seconds, but it's so worth doing it properly.

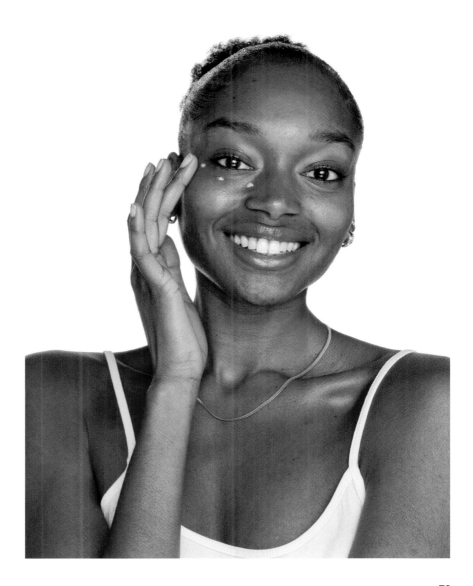

Concealer

Once you've neutralised the shadows under your eyes with corrector, it's time to place your concealer on top.

Being able to conceal what we perceive to be imperfections can be hugely helpful, especially if said 'imperfection' is getting you down. Thankfully, concealer can minimise, if not completely banish, the appearance of scars, spots, dark circles, melasma and even tattoos.

APPLICATION

I like to place the concealer directly on top of the corrector and then use my ring finger (or brush, depending on your preference) to press the concealer into the skin. Start in the inner corner of the eye, then work your way out towards the outer corner. The concealer will be at its most intense where you lay the product down, but when you pat the concealer out towards the outer corner of the eye, the coverage will naturally be

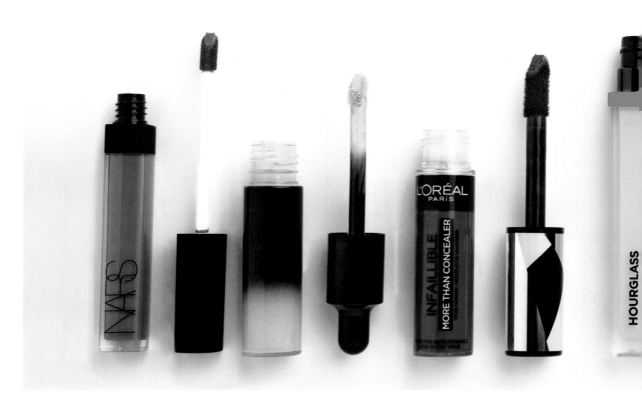

less as you're simply removing the excess concealer. Take your time when pressing the concealer into place, it may take a few moments; making sure the product is well worked into the skin rather than sitting on the surface in a thick layer really does help prevent the concealer from creasing.

EQUIPMENT

There are a few tools such as concealer brushes, sponges and clean fingers. Flat concealer brushes are excellent for laying the product onto the skin. Round, domed brushes are ideal for buffing and blending concealer into the skin. Just like with foundation, the softer the brush you use to apply your concealer, the lighter the finish. The more dense the brush, the fuller the coverage.

Some concealers are quite tacky in texture, which isn't always a bad thing – it can prevent concealer from looking dry – but it may be necessary to set these formulas with a bit of powder, which will extend the wear of your concealer.

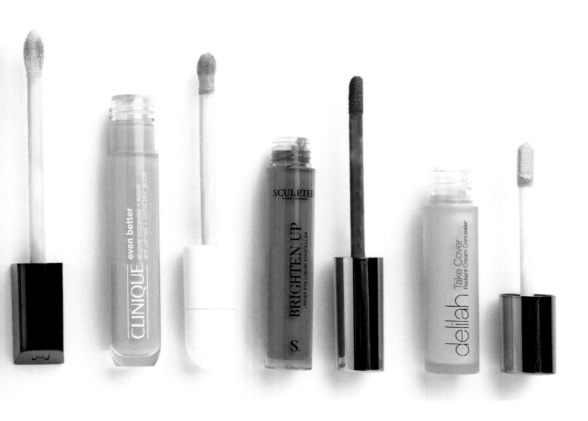

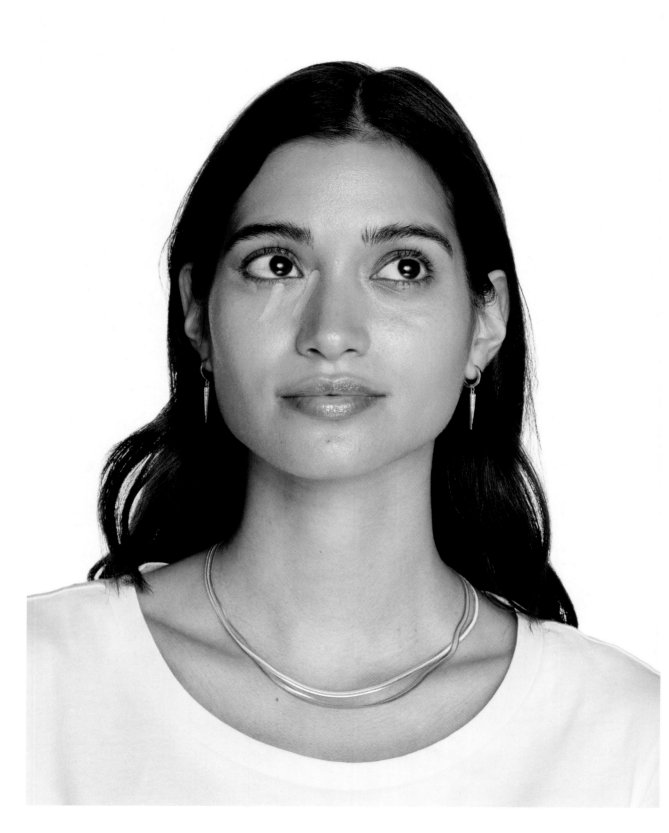

I suggest a loose powder for setting the under eye. Just a tiny bit on a fluffy brush will set the makeup in place or use a velvet powder puff to completely mattify – just be sure to have pressed out any creases before you apply the powder as you don't want to set a concealer crease in place inadvertently.

Under eye concealer can also work wonders for further toning down or controlling redness in the skin, namely on the top of the cheeks. If this is something you struggle with, tap your concealer both out towards the outer corner of the eye and down onto the top of the cheeks to further control and eliminate redness in the cheeks. This makes under eye concealer more natural looking and helps it blend with the rest of the base compared to when it is only applied directly under the eyes.

UNDER EYE BAKING

There has been a big trend on social media for baking under eye concealer in the last few years.

Baking is the process of applying a generous amount of light loose powder on top of your concealer and allowing it to set into, and be absorbed by, the makeup. You leave the powder to settle for a while before dusting away the excess. It is very effective for locking concealer in place, mattifying and even brightening your concealer if you use a very bright powder. However, it's not at all flattering in real life for those who have a few lines around the eyes. It can make the skin look dry and can exacerbate the appearance of lines, making them even more pronounced. Of course, it's an aesthetic that many love and lots of people don't struggle with fine lines and wrinkles around the eyes, but if you do, I would approach this technique with caution! If you're using a more matte finish concealer, setting with loose powder isn't always necessary.

CONCEALERS I LIKE:

Lightweight:
– RMS Beauty UnCoverup
– Bobbi Brown Intensive Serum Foundation
– Armani Luminous Silk Concealer
– e.l.f. Hydrating Camo Concealer
– IT Cosmetics Bye Bye Under Eye

Medium coverage:
– Bobbi Brown Skin Concealer Stick
– Charlotte Tilbury Magic Away
– Urban Decay Stay Naked Concealer
– Clé de Peau Beauté Concealer
– Anastasia Beverly Hills Magic Touch Concealer

Full coverage:
– L'Oréal Infallible More Than Concealer
– Nars Radiant Creamy Concealer
– MAC Studio Fix
– Tarte Shape Tape
– Huda Beauty FauxFilter Luminous Matte Concealer

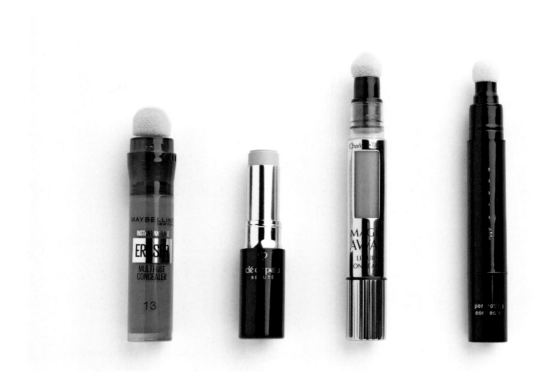

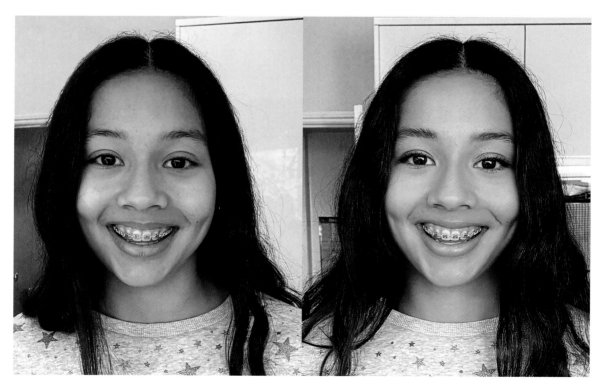

Tweaking

Concealer is the number one thing I will tweak. If you are ever getting ready for an event and you want your makeup to be just so, photograph it. You can take a selfie in lots of different lights and it allows you to quickly ascertain how the makeup is translating and identify if there's anything that needs changing. Check:

· **Concealer** I apply a bit to the top of the cheeks where the under eye and cheek meet if the blush has been placed a bit too high.

· **Powder** I apply this if I can see any hotspots that look a bit shiny.

· **Bronzer** I might apply a bit more bronzer if the base is looking pale.

· **Eyeliner** I will soften the lower lash liner if it's looking too slim, which can make it look a bit harsh.

· **Blush** I'll often add a bit more blush. I'm always cautious not to overdo it, but if it is too insipid it can look a bit flat. The shade doesn't necessarily need to be bright. Often it just needs to be a bit stronger, which you can quickly achieve by adding a touch more.

Teenage beauty

What each teenager considers to be 'age-appropriate makeup' is totally subjective. Whilst Natural Collection Clear mascara and Blistex lip balm was my makeup routine as a 14-year-old, today some young people go to school in what I would consider full makeup. It's best not to overcomplicate skincare for young people as a simple routine is so important. The number one rule when wearing makeup is that it must be removed properly. Below are the items I recommend for young people just starting to wear makeup.

Makeup Remover – A micellar water is a great choice for quick and easy makeup removal before cleansing. Apply to a reusable cotton pad and sweep over the complexion and hold over any eye makeup. Sweep gently to remove. I like the Simple and Bioderma micellar waters.

Cleanser – Remove any remaining makeup or micellar water residue on the skin with a cleanser like CeraVe Hydrating Cleanser or La Roche-Posay Toleriane Foaming Gel Wash. If you are struggling with spots, then a cleanser that contains salicylic acid can be beneficial. The entire Effaclar range from La Roche-Posay is excellent for acne-prone skin but you can also use Eucerin, CeraVe and Cetaphil.

Moisturiser – I always recommend light and simple when it comes to moisturiser for young people. Something like Simple Kind To Skin Moisturising Lotion or CeraVe Facial Moisturising Lotion is great, followed by SPF such as La Roche-Posay Anthelios.

Tinted Moisturiser – Use a great lightweight base option, something like Erborian BB cream or Rimmel Kind and Free Moisturising Skin Tint.

Concealer – Keep in a bag or pencil case if spots are a problem. I'll sound like a broken record here but L'Oréal Infallible is an excellent concealer for teens – a tiny bit under the eye is great for brightening dark circles, but it also offers brilliant coverage for blemishes.

Cream Blush – Yes, I love cream blush on young skin. It is quick and easy to apply and looks natural. Glossier Cloud Paints are gorgeous, as are the Max Factor Miracle Touch Creamy Blushers.

Brow Gel – I didn't start filling in my brows until I was in my late twenties but brows have been major in beauty the last few years, so a brow pencil is a must for many. Start by using clear brow gel, for example Got2b Glued 4 Brows or e.l.f. Cosmetics Wow Brow Gel.

Mascara – I recommend using Maybelline Lash Sensation Sky High Mascara or L'Oréal Telescopic.

Lip Gloss – I cherished my Natural Collection Clear Lip Gloss when I was a teenager. It would go all sticky at the top, get passed round my class mates and become cloudy over time, but it was so treasured! Now there are so many gorgeous affordable glosses out there but you can't go wrong with the likes of NYX, Revolution, e.l.f., Rimmel London, Primark, Maybelline and Kiko Milano.

Disguising Pores

I'm asked about how to disguise pores all the time. The jury is still out when it comes to whether or not you can shrink pore size, but you can absolutely help by clearing out any dirt or debris that may be clogging your pores and making them look bigger.

Now, I'm not a skincare expert, but I do know that salicylic acid is a go-to for pore clearing and is recommended for those looking to treat, or even prevent, break-outs. It gently exfoliates the skin and breaks down oils that can clog pores. It comes in an array of different guises: in face washes, creams, serums and treatments.

Other helpful and preventative ingredients include glycolic acid, lactic acid and niacinamide.

When it comes to makeup prep and makeup itself, there are a few things you can do. Before applying the base, you can use a **pore minimising cream**, most of which contain little spherical silicone particles that will fill in and disguise any large pores, as well as create a blurring effect, which is more of an optical illusion that will soften their appearance.

Setting powders help enormously too as they will gently dry down any wet makeup, which, if glistening in the light, may highlight open pores. Some powders are designed with pores in mind and contain silica, again to blur the appearance of open pores and absorb excess oil that may come through makeup.

If you're concerned about pore size don't think that you're limited to only oil-free matte makeup. You don't want to add too much glow or highlighter, especially to larger pores you are trying to disguise, but you can wear illuminating makeup in the areas that don't have any large pores and then simply mattify the areas that do. For example, you could prep your skin with a pore-minimising primer through the T-zone and front of the cheeks and apply an illuminating tinted moisturiser to the outer corners of the face. Then use a concealer for the under eyes and areas of concern, and set the T-zone with a pore-minimising powder. Use a highlighter on other areas, like the very top of the brow bone, the cupid's bow or the top of the bridge of the nose.

*

Salicylic acid: Salicylic acid is organic and a beta-hydroxy acid (BHA) used to help target and exfoliate pore congestion and dull skin.

THE BASE: POWDER

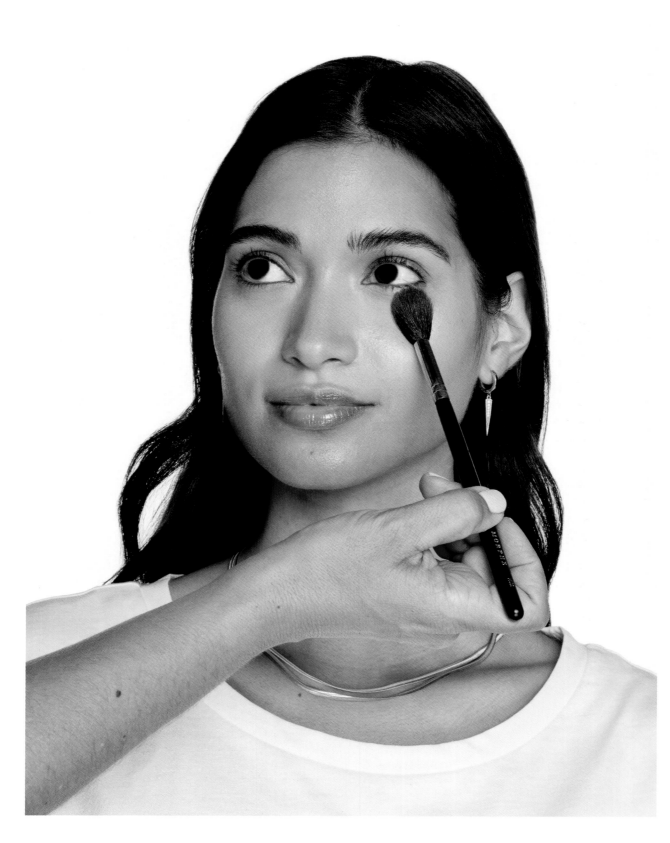

THE BASE: POWDER

| *Powder has gathered a bit of a bad reputation in recent years, with makeup trends leaning to the more dewy finish.*

There has also been a little scaremongering from the beauty press that powder can make the skin look dull or more mature, as well as a healthy amount of confusion over the purpose of powder as a setting agent, with the introduction of many setting sprays (see page 90).

Throughout history, the makeup powders that have been used haven't always been good for the skin. Dated as far back as 2000 BC, toxic face powder and kohl eyeliner were found in ancient tombs and we know that Queen Elizabeth I wore a lot of heavy, white face powder to hide her smallpox scars and because bright, light skin was a sign of good health (and fertility, I believe). However, this powder was full of lead, which some believe contributed to her eventual blood poisoning. Not exactly what we want from our makeup!

From the toxic makeup powders of ancient Egypt to the more commercially available makeup of the last century, powder has evolved dramatically. Eventually the ingredients of makeup were regulated and the use of lead prohibited. However, the appearance of face powder even up to the late 80s and early 90s was still quite heavy.

Most of us will have a memory of an older relative who had a big tub of loose powder and a huge powder puff, whose finishing touch to their beauty routine would create billowing puffs of powder. Perhaps, like me, you had a parent whose skin smelled of powder or can remember that familiar sound of a compact powder sponge sweeping across the skin to rid it of any shine. Three things my mum always did at the end of a long car journey to herald we were nearly at our final destination were a slick of lipstick, a sweep of powder and a few spritzes of perfume . . . I digress.

My point is that the skin of those who wore powder often did look very matte, even dry. You could sometimes see the powder caught in the fine downy hair on the skin. It didn't help skin glow, so when the rise in popularity of luminous, dewy skin came around, many believed they needed to ditch their powder altogether.

*
Quick side note:
If you are interested in the history of makeup, two books that I highly recommend are *Timeless* by Louise Young and Lisa Eldridge's *Face Paint*. They are both absolutely fascinating.

Powders today

Powders have never been as finely milled as they are now or have more skin-loving ingredients.

Talc-free to pure minerals to oil-free to moisturising to light-reflecting, fine-line blurring, there are literally hundreds to choose from.

The most notable difference in modern powders is how finely milled they are – teeny tiny particles you can barely see but feel silky between your fingers. These can set makeup without any of the potentially skin-ageing finishes of less-modern powders. There are even powders available that contain key moisturising ingredients, like hyaluronic acid, to prevent them looking and feeling dry. Admittedly, application has evolved too, from the previously used large face puffs to delicate brushes and sponges, so you have much more control over where the powder is placed.

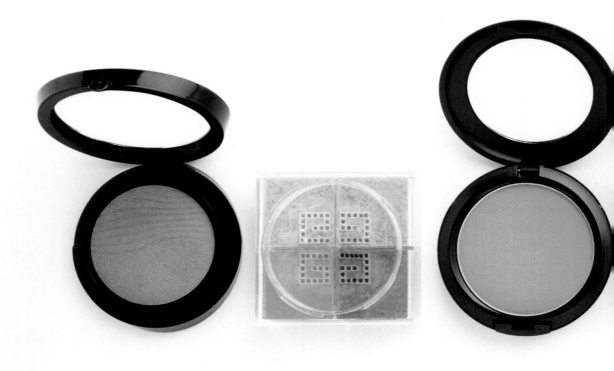

Setting makeup

To set makeup, I highly recommend the use of a **translucent loose powder**. Translucent means it doesn't hold any/much coloured pigment. You can, of course, buy skin-toned powders, however, I prefer to use translucent powders as sometimes if a pigmented powder is applied to set a liquid foundation, the powder can oxidise when it comes into contact with the oils in the foundation.

What that means is that as the powder sets into and dries the foundation, the shade of the powder intensifies and turns a deeper shade, thus making your base makeup look darker than intended. It is particularly important that you use translucent powder under the eyes for this very reason. You don't want to ruin all the work you've done brightening your under eye by using too dark a powder to set it.

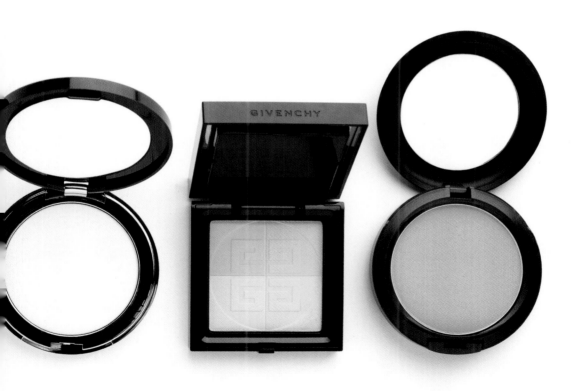

GETTING A NATURAL FINISH WITH POWDER

It's probably worth noting at this point that for the most natural finish, you want to ensure you don't have any excess foundation on the skin before applying your powder. For example, when working with my clients I always start with base makeup, but I don't set it with powder until the makeup is almost completely finished. This gives the base products time to settle into the skin and dry a little. It also means I can go back to the base and perfect any areas that need a bit more coverage, or blend out any creases.

APPLICATION

1   I highly recommend taking a clean base brush (a synthetic foundation buffing brush, of sorts – just don't use anything too firm as you may move the makeup underneath) and use it to gently sweep over the base makeup. This will help to diffuse and blend any edges and remove any excess product.

2   Apply powder. I like to use a small fluffy brush first to sweep the powder through the T-zone – the area where most of us have slightly larger pores that secrete sebum (oil). Oil isn't the enemy, not at all. The skin needs oil to protect it, but it is the oil that can cause makeup to become shiny or move, so that's why I focus powder in those areas.

For a more matte finish, use a sponge or a velvet powder puff as they lay more product on the skin than a brush. Dip the applicator into the powder, remove any excess by tapping the sponge/puff into the palm of your hand, then press into the areas you wish to mattify. Be methodical with your powder placement to ensure the matte finish is seamless and not blotchy. For example, I press a sponge using light taps, working from the centre of my forehead out towards my temple, then repeat on the other side instead of simply randomly blotting in the area.

The powder helps to dry the surface of the makeup and essentially creates a seal that is harder for the oils to penetrate. Without powder, base makeup will dry to the air, which is fine, but as soon as your sebaceous glands start producing oil and it seeps out through the pores, it will be absorbed by the makeup, which will become wet looking.

- As a general rule of thumb, **if you have oily skin** and don't want too much shine through the centre of your face, then look to use an **oil-free powder or one that contains silica,** so it can help absorb any excess oil.

- **If your skin is on the dry side**, then a **moisturising powder** is the obvious choice.

Powders can contain oil and if you're hoping to banish shine from your face, then you're going to want to avoid oil in your setting powder. Similarly, if you struggle to keep your skin hydrated, you're going to want to avoid any moisture-drinking ingredients like silica, which could make your skin look drier.

What is the T-zone?

The T-zone is the centre of the forehead, above the eyebrows, between the eyebrows, around the nose, front of the cheek, upper lip and chin.

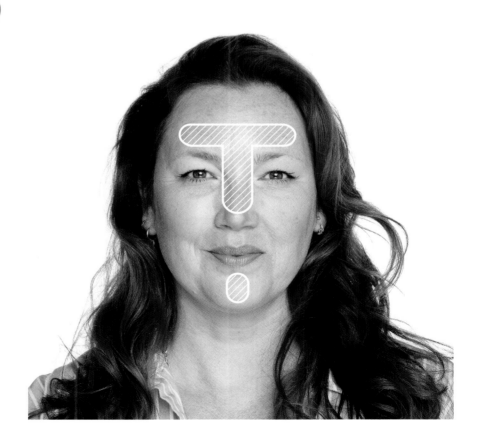

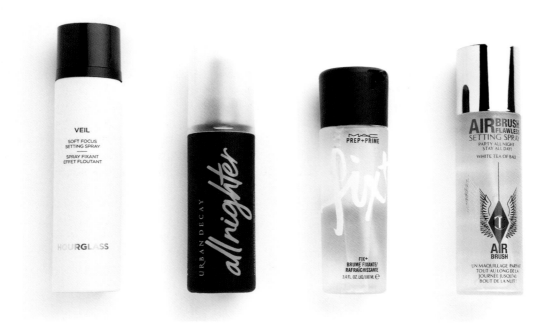

Setting sprays

There are many on the market these days with lots of different key focuses:

· To rehydrate your makeup, thus reviving tired-looking makeup
  (perfect for those with naturally dry or dehydrated skin).
· To add shimmer.
· To control oil.
· To mattify.
· To prolong the wear of makeup.

It's easy to mistake a rehydrating spray for a setting spray as many rehydrating sprays are called setting sprays – confusing, I know.

By using either, you are adding both water and oil to your makeup. This is great if you have dry skin and you feel makeup exacerbates that, but if you have oily skin or are looking for a spray to prolong the wear of your makeup, then you must use a powder first.

> *Setting sprays don't compare in the efficiency stakes to setting powders.*

For makeup to be long-wearing, apply your powder as suggested above, then spritz with a specific long-wearing setting spray.

As always, I'll list the setting sprays I use most and their benefits, but I'll say here that by far the most effective setting spray I keep in my kit is **Urban Decay All Nighter**. There are lots of incarnations of this iconic spray, but I prefer to use the original. It really does hold makeup in place and will waterproof your makeup to the point of you being able to jump into a pool and it won't move – it's that good. I don't use it every day, however. The old-school MUA in me still likes to let my skin 'breathe', so I only use it on myself when I really need that longevity from my makeup.

It seems lots of us have been led to believe that you can use a spray in place of powder. Many of us therefore have inadvertently been adding unwanted, unnecessary moisture to our makeup, leading to frustration when makeup doesn't in fact stay in place.

BAKING

As mentioned in under eyes (page 77), loose powder is also used to bake makeup – the practice that originated in drag to set liquid bases in place and brighten, most commonly under the eyes, and either side of the nose and below the cheek to sharpen the contour.

Usually applied with a damp sponge, you place a lot of loose powder onto the area in question and allow it to 'bake' for a good 10–15 minutes before sweeping away the excess powder. In that time, the powder will be absorbed by the concealer or foundation and indeed 'lock' the makeup in place.

The only thing to be wary of is that this technique can dry out the skin and make fine lines look even more pronounced, so if you are at all concerned about fine lines, I would not recommend this.

I really like to sharpen my contour under my cheekbones by baking the area with a lighter powder, so that's something I'll do more often, but I prefer a lighter powder application under my eyes.

COLOUR & WARMTH: BRONZER & CONTOUR

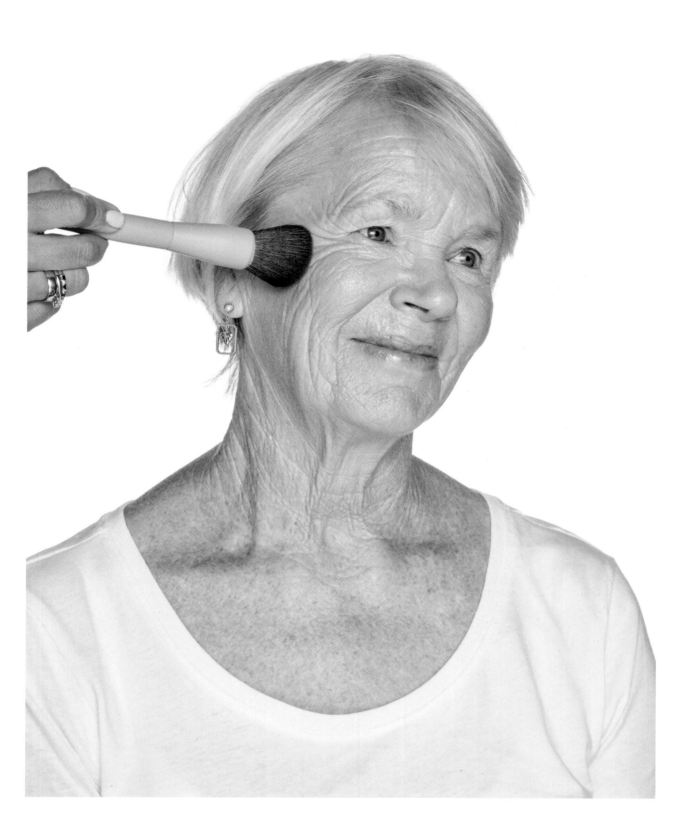

BRONZER

> *I am unashamed of my obsession with bronzer.*
> *I absolutely love it.*

I often encounter people who think bronzer is only for those wanting to look tanned, but I use bronzer on most people to shade and shape the face, no matter the skin tone.

Choosing the right bronzer

When it comes to which bronzer to choose for your skin tone, it's not as tricky as you might think. Simply look to see what you notice in your skin. Is there a yellowish/golden tone? Or is there more pinkish/red?

· **If you can detect golden/yellow tones**, then it's likely you'd naturally tan more of a golden shade, which would mean you'd suit **a more golden-toned bronzer**.

· **If you can detect a bit more red in the skin**, it's probable that you tan more of a reddish tone, in which case, **a bronzer with a bit more red** will suit you best.

· **If you can't detect any gold or any red**, then you probably have a neutral undertone, in which case **a pinkish/brown bronzer** is probably better, as too much gold or red could look unnatural.

I recommend a matte bronzer for every day rather than a sparkly one as you don't necessarily want shimmer in the daytime, especially if using bronzer to contour and shade the face. You can always add sparkle in the areas where you want to glimmer once your makeup is done.

**GEL BRONZER
I LIKE:**

– Clinique Sun-Kissed Face Gelee

– Iconic London Sheer Bronze

– Drunk Elephant D-Bronzi Drops

– Chantecaille Radiance Gel Bronzer

– Milk Makeup Bionic Bronzer

**CREAM BRONZER
I LIKE:**

– Huda Beauty Tantour

– Chanel Les Beiges Healthy Glow Bronzing Cream

– e.l.f. Cosmetics Putty Bronzer

– Nars Laguna Bronzing Cream

– Fenty Beauty Cheeks Out Freestyle Cream Bronzer

– Anastasia Beverly Hills Cream Bronzer

BRONZER FOR FAIR COMPLEXIONS

The only people who I might not use bronzer on are those with porcelain skin, who wouldn't naturally tan, because adding a brownish tone to their skin doesn't always look natural.

For those with very fair skin, instead use a pinkish tone or a blush in the areas you would typically use bronzer. It has a very similar effect when trying to add a bit of dimension or look sun-kissed. You cannot use this for contouring, however. If you are looking to contour, then stick to a light greyish contour tone.

I use bronzer on all skin tones. The only exception being if someone has a very deep skin tone, then I might use highlighter to almost 'reverse contour' – I focus on adding light to the top of the cheeks and bridge of the nose to amplify the face contours instead of shading below the cheek or either side of the nose.

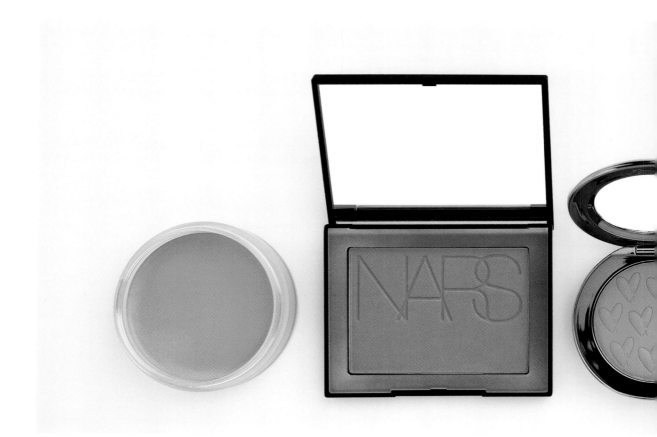

EQUIPMENT

I suggest using a small brush to contour and a large brush to bronze.

With contouring, a smaller brush helps because you're looking to achieve a slightly sharper, more condensed application. You don't want to diffuse too much colour over too great an area or you'll lose the effect you're hoping to create.

> *With bronzer, it's key to have it looking seamless and totally diffused, as if it is how your skin looks naturally. I find a larger, slightly flatter brush can help to achieve that.*

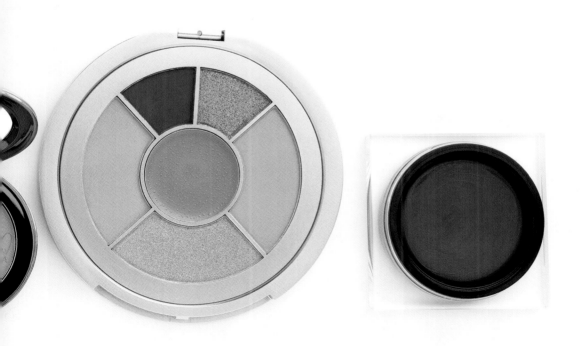

BRUSH TECHNIQUE

When you've dipped your brush into your bronzer, be sure to tap the head of the brush by lightly pressing it into the palm of your hand. I know lots of people simply tap their brush, but I find this means the pigment drops off and you lose it from the bristles. By tapping the brush into your palm, you are pushing the pigment into the brush between the bristles and storing it within its head so that as you sweep over the face you:

a) Don't get a big blob of pigment, which can happen if you have lots of bronzer sitting on the tip of your brush bristles.
b) You can layer and build the colour as you sweep.

PLACEMENT

A little bronzer won't necessarily make you look like you've been on holiday, but it will make your face appear more dimensional.

So, let's start with placement before we get into texture. Bronzer is amazing for helping to add shape to the face, especially after foundation application, which can leave the face looking a little flat and a single tone.

As a basic rule, I recommend applying bronzer to the higher points of the face, so the top of the forehead and the temples, top of the cheekbones, top of the nose, top of the ears and any excess from the brush down the neck. This will instantly create depth and shape and warm the skin around the edges, much like safe sun exposure would. For those with shallow foreheads, you don't always need to bronze your forehead if you don't naturally tan there, but for those with higher foreheads, it's a great way of subtly disguising the size of the forehead.

If your bronzer is looking a little 'stripy' for whatever reason, simply blend out the edges with a clean brush to soften.

For a more sun-kissed look, simply use more bronzer – it's really that simple.

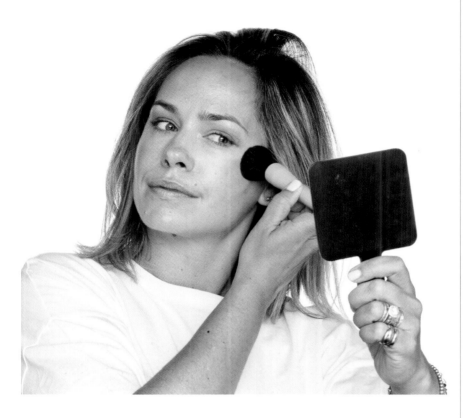

If you have the right shade of bronzer for your skin tone, you don't necessarily need to use a darker one when you have a tan, just a bit more of the one you already have.

I mention using bronzer on the neck because many people find their neck is naturally fairer than the rest of their body, as it's shaded by the jawline. So to make sure the face, neck and decollate are the same tone, sweep your bronzer down your neck and onto the chest too if necessary.

If you are wearing your hair up and have bronzed your face, be sure to take your bronzer behind the ears and over the back of the neck, if necessary, so you're not left with unwanted light patches.

Some find that their face is lighter than their chest due to more fervent use of sun protection. If this is the case, this is where using bronzer as a corrector is really useful. Still matching your foundation to the colour of your skin, use bronzer to warm the edges enough to match the tone of the skin on your chest. If it's the other way around, you may need to warm the neck and chest to ensure synergy with your skin tone.

CONTOUR

Bronzer can also be used to contour the face. Contour means using makeup, both dark and light, to create shadows and highlight to define and sculpt the face.

This is a technique that has been used since makeup was first invented. It was perfected in the days of early black-and-white film but has had a major resurgence in mainstream popularity in recent years thanks to reality TV stars, social media and what we call 'Instagram makeup'.

Contouring can be magic. Artists like the late Kevyn Aucoin and, more recently, Alexis Stone use contouring to completely alter their or their clients' appearance to resemble others.

A tighter-bound, flat, round-headed brush can be useful when contouring as the firmness of the brush means the placement of product is both intense and exactly where you want it. The brush won't spread the colour too far, meaning you have total control over where the contour shade is. It's then up to you how you blend it. If you use a fluffier brush, the product will disperse and you won't achieve the sharpness desired.

While contouring has the ability to be completely transformative, it doesn't have to be dramatic.

It's the subtle shaping effect of bronzing that makes me feel most 'me'. The shading around the edges of the face gives my complexion life, and the subtle shading below my cheekbones gives my face more structure. In reality, I have quite a flat face. Bronzing the top of my forehead helps to reduce the appearance of its length. The contour through the crease of my eye makes me feel polished when I am not wearing any other eye makeup and the touch of contour down the sides of my nose makes me less self-conscious about the bump in it.

However, I never look 'contoured' in the way we've become familiar with in recent years, as it's always blended out and so not too strong. That doesn't mean I don't appreciate stronger contouring – I really could watch others contour their faces for hours – it's just not a look that I love on myself.

Where to contour for your face shape

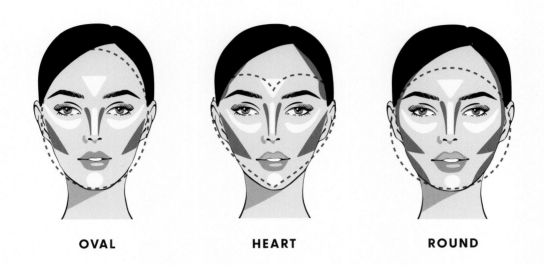

OVAL   HEART   ROUND

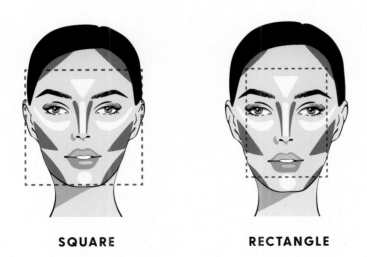

SQUARE   RECTANGLE

Finding what you love

One of my 'ah ha' moments came as I sat on the floor of Blackwell's bookshop in Oxford as a student and was transfixed by an image of Gwyneth Paltrow in Kevyn's book *Face Forward*, made up to look like James Dean. The likeness was uncanny and it was the first time I think I really appreciated the power of how makeup can transform. I eventually bought the much-thumbed book and another 'ah ha' moment came when my housemate Liz looked over my shoulder as I studied another two faces in the book: this time Chandra North and Isabella Rossellini.

I was mesmerised by the two faces and the power of two tiny tweaks to each. Isabella is over a double-page spread. On one page her brows are soft and subtly filled in, on the other they are brushed up and spiked. This small change completely transforms the look and feel of the image.

On the next page, Chandra again has identical makeup on each page bar her lip shape. On one side, Kevyn has rounded and softened the lip shape and on the other he has made a real point of the cupid's bow. Again, this tiny difference makes all the difference. With the more tinted lip, Chandra looks more pixie and elfin.

I was flicking between the two pages in awe for the longest time and Liz simply said, 'You really do love makeup, don't you Hannah?' and I realised I did.

I didn't just like makeup or enjoy makeup, I loved it and everything about it. It was a really significant turning point in the whole trajectory of my life and career.

There is an assumption that contouring can look fake or heavy, when that really isn't the case.

· The key areas that I most like to contour are **the forehead, the temples, the crease of the eyes, the nose, cheekbones and jawline.**

· By **shading below the cheekbones**, you create a shadow, making it look like the face recedes or is sunken a little in that area to **give the illusion of more prominent cheekbones.**

· If you **shade along the jawline**, you can **sharpen its appearance** and disguise the neck by shading it.

*

Hue:
The colour or shade.

SHADES

Contour shades are traditionally a little more flat than bronzing shades as their purpose is to create the illusion of shadow rather than warming the skin.

Bronzers usually have a golden or red hue, whereas contour shades are more neutral, varying from light grey in colour for porcelain skin tones through to deep, flat brown for black and brown skin tones. These tones can look a little ashy on the skin if not used correctly, so as a general rule of thumb I use both: contour below the feature and bronzer above.

The greyish hue should create the shadow and the bronzer shades should create the warmth. However, there's no hard and fast rule to what order you do this in.

APPLICATION

Generally speaking, to help emphasise the appearance of cheekbones, you want to apply your contour shade just below the cheekbone.

1 If you're unsure where that is on your face, roll the handle of a makeup brush or a pen down the side of your face until you feel it sit under the cheekbone. If you press it gently in place and then lift off, you should be able to see a slight imprint on the skin, and that is where you should focus your contour.

2 Next, simply draw your contour along that line until you reach the outer corner of your iris when looking straight ahead. I generally don't bring cheek contour any further in towards the centre of the face as I find this can add unwanted shade and make blush look a bit flat, so just be cautious not to bring your contour too far forward.

3 Once you have applied the contour shade, gently blend upwards to soften the edges. I don't recommend blending down as this could make your contour shade look too low. You want the shade beneath the contour to be true to your skin tone.

However, if you're wanting to create the illusion of a higher cheekbone, you can place your contour higher up the cheekbone and highlight the very highest point.

4 When contouring the nose, usually people are trying to make it look slimmer by shading the sides and highlighting the bridge. The closer together you make the shades either side of the nose, the narrower you will make it appear. Of course, no one 'needs' a nose slimmer than the one they're born with, but it's a technique one can use if you so wish.

You can also use contour around the tip of the nose to make it look more rounded. Alternatively, create the illusion of a button nose by shading the underside of the tip and drawing a line in a contour colour across the nose where you'd like to create the illusion of a slight upturn, roughly a third of the way up usually.

'BAKING' CONTOUR

If your contour shade is too deep on either side of your nose, then you may inadvertently make the base look wider. To avoid this, lots of people 'bake' either side of their nose contour. This is a technique whereby you press, usually with a sponge, a condensed amount of light loose powder along the sides of the nose below the contour colour and leave it to sit on the skin or 'bake', as the technique name would suggest. This allows the foundation to absorb some of the powder and brighten in the area applied, ensuring the base of the sides of your nose are indeed light and not too dark, eliminating the risk of making the base look wider.

Again, blending is absolutely key, so I recommend using a much smaller brush for perfecting nose contour – a slim eyeshadow brush is usually what I reach for so you can create slim lines that you can easily blend. If your 'tool' is too big, your shading will be over-exaggerated and clunky and that can contribute to your contour looking unnatural.

When it comes to the rest of your contour, you don't need as small a brush for the cheeks, temple and jawline and you can use the same brush for each. I use a mid-size contouring brush, usually called a face shading brush, or the edge of my foundation brush if I'm in a rush.

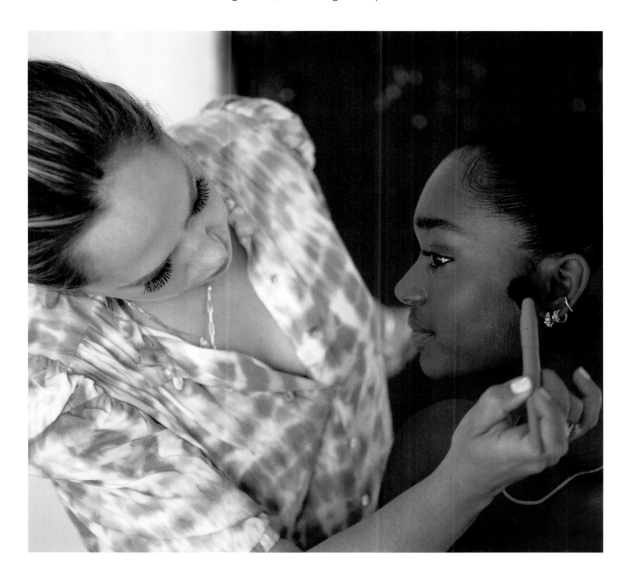

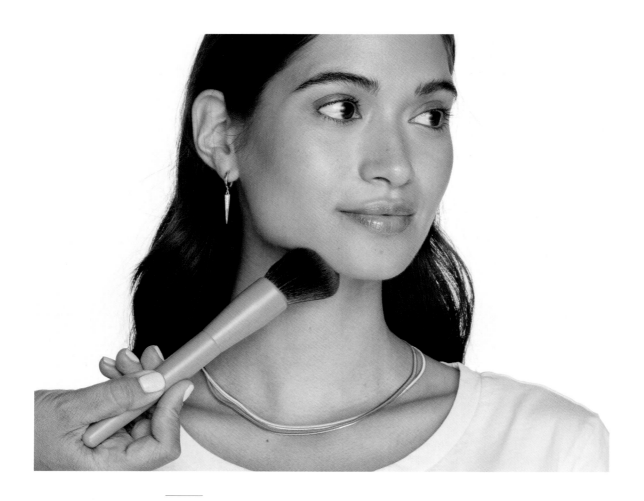

WHICH TEXTURE?

You can get bronzing and contouring products in a number of different textures, namely creams and powders, but you can also get bronzing gels. I'm particularly keen on the gels for creating really natural bronzed looks without adding too much makeup to the skin.

· **A gel works best when using a lightweight base** as it's fairly 'wet' and can move heavier foundations. It's great if you're wearing something like a tinted moisturiser or BB cream.

· If you like to wear **a base with a bit more pigment and more coverage**, then you're **best choosing between a cream or powder**.

· If your **skin is on the oily side**, you may wish to just use **powder** so you're not adding too much cream to the skin.

- Likewise, if your **skin is on the dry side**, then it makes sense to look to **cream-based bronzer and contour products**.

I tend to use both cream and powder on most of my clients. I particularly like to build up the bronzer lightly with cream-based products worked into the foundation before I set it, sometimes with cream bronzers, sometimes simply using deeper foundation or concealer shades. I then set the colour in place with powder versions.

> *You might think that could look heavy, but I have always worked on the principle of building lots of light layers to create beautiful-looking, long-wearing makeup.*

APPLICATION

I carry with me in my kit foundation palettes (the Bobbi Brown Cosmetics BBU is a kit must-have, but I also make my own by decanting into empty palettes), so I can mix and blend on the job, combining shades to create a client's perfect bronzing or contour shade. I also carry specific contour palettes for that slightly flatter tone.

I find that blending cream into cream (bronzer into base) creates the most flattering natural finish. I recommend cream bronzers first that you can let 'sit and set' while you do the rest of your makeup. Then when I start setting makeup with powder, I'll perfect the base and set using a combination of translucent powder in the areas I want to keep bright and bronzers and contour powders in areas where I want to maintain shade.

REVERSE CONTOUR

I recently learnt a variation on this technique during a masterclass with makeup artist Joy Adenuga. A 'reverse contour' used on her clients with black skin, where she simply and very finely highlights the centre of the nose from just below the inner corner of the eyes to the tip with highlighter. This bounces light and brings the centre of the nose to the forefront rather than shading the sides of the nose and it works brilliantly.

COLOUR & WARMTH: BLUSH

BLUSH

Oh, how I love blush. A flush of blush to the apples of the cheek instantly adds life and energy to every face.

My feeling is not universally shared, however. I know lots of people who are nervous of blush and have clients who forbid me from applying it (true story).

If I am met with resistance or reluctance from clients, I will always endeavour to encourage the use of blush because I believe it to be so flattering. You're essentially looking to replicate the appearance of the cheeks when they flush with colour after exercise and, much like bronzer, the aim is to put colour back into the face that base makeup may have neutralised.

It's different when it comes to fashion and, say, a designer doesn't want blush on the models for their show or look book. In fact, it can often be that the designer doesn't want any colour in a model's face whatsoever (usually to let the clothes do all the talking).

I did have an interesting encounter with a well-known designer recently. They were styling one of my brides and they suggested there was too much blush. So reluctant was I to tone it down, that I did my best to fake toning it down! When you're wearing a pale colour from head to toe, it can drain the face of colour and wash the wearer out, so a little blush maintains a healthy finish to the skin. Whilst no cross words were uttered, it was an interesting moment when creative opinions differ!

TONE DOWN

A tone down is something I will do if I see my makeup in the monitor or from a distance and feel the colour is too strong. I simply blend some of the makeup away with a clean brush.

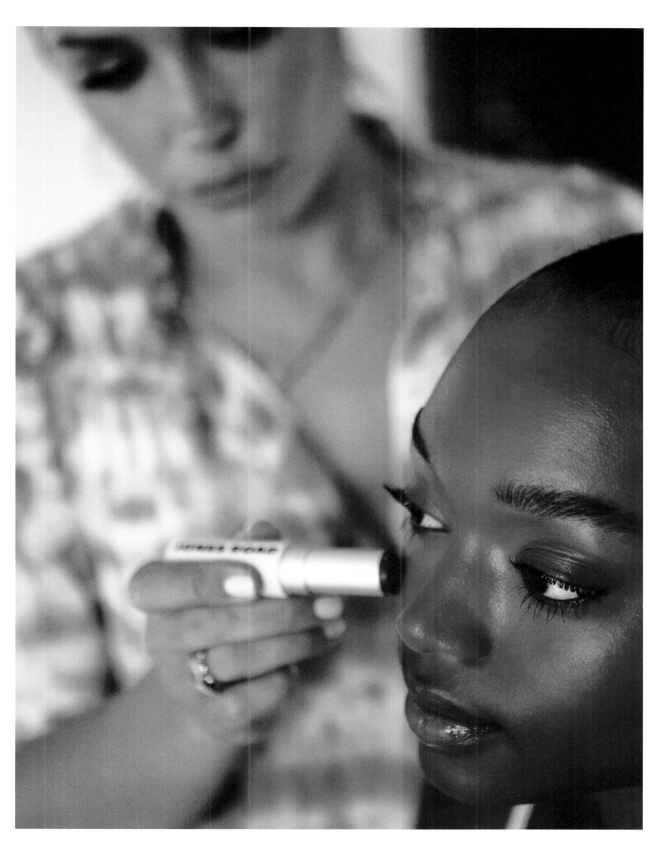

WHICH COLOUR?

You can use a whole array of colours when it comes to blush, and in a number of different textures, depending on the finish you're hoping to create.

> *I've always believed that a bright, blue-based pink blush looks incredible on everyone.*

Used lightly on pale skin tones and layered for more intensity on black skin, a blue-based pink blush never fails to look good.

That doesn't mean to say that everyone will like pink blush. I know many have an aversion to pink altogether, but that's where other colour blushes come into play. From pale peach to brown to pink to red to plum, there are literally hundreds of shades available.

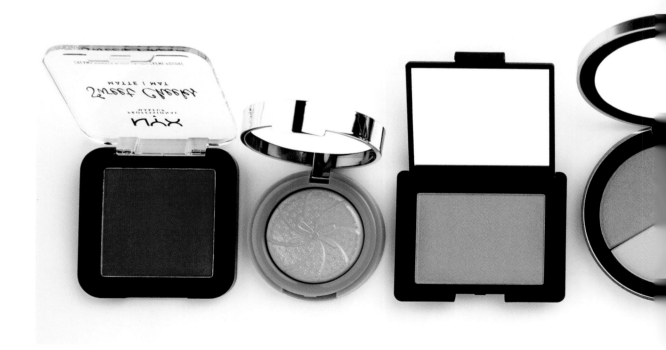

Whilst there are no set rules to guide colour choice (I'm a huge believer in the 'if you love it, go for it' mentality when it comes to makeup colours), there are shades I gravitate towards for different skin tones:

· I often encounter people with **very fair skin who have been led to believe they can only wear muted coral tones.** While, yes, muted coral tones look stunning on porcelain skin tones, so do pinks and plums. Even reds! A deep cherry red that some might assume was most suited to black skin (and, yes, I love deep cherry blush on black skin too) can look exquisite on fair skin. Think lightweight base, glossy eyes, full lashes, fluffy brushed-up brows and a clear gloss lip – can you see how gorgeous that would be?!

· **Pinky corals** look incredible on **olive and brown skin tones**.

· **Deep plums, berries and oranges** are stunning on **black skin**.

As I said, these are preferences, not rules. I will always be led by whatever colour inspires me or suits the colour harmony of the outfit.

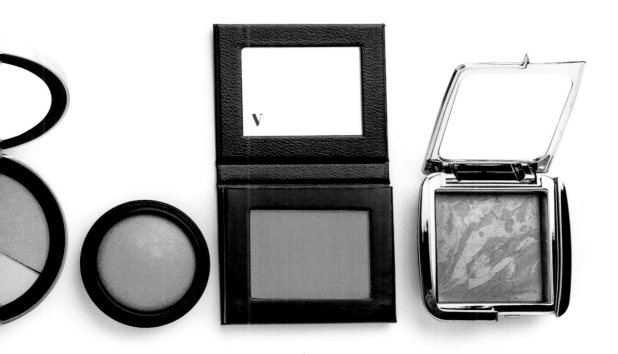

APPLICATION

Placement can also vary depending on the style you're looking to create. I have always loved blush placed high on the apples of the cheek. If you're not sure where that is, it's the centre of the part of the cheek that rises when you smile. I will always ask my clients to smile to help me find where to start with blush.

Blush trends

Blush swept over the tops of the apples of the cheeks and blended back to meet the bronzer is the most 'classic' of application styles as it pretty much emulates that natural flushed look one gets after a brisk walk (or whatever gets your heart rate going). Saying that, blush trends do tend to come and go:

Think of **draping**, for example, a style really popular in the 80s, where blush was placed high on the top of the cheekbones and blended up through the temples and into the crease of the eye (Blondie, Madonna and Boy George were fans). Essentially contouring but with blush.

More recently, the **Igari** trend, originating in Japan, became a 'thing' on social media. This is when blush is placed high, right under the eyes and across the nose, to mimic the flush one might get after drinking alcohol, earning it the name 'drunk blush'.

Or there's the **sun-kissed** trend, where blush is added to the chin, nose and forehead as well as the cheeks.

Right now, there's a movement for creating more of a **'lifted' look** with your blush, so heading back to the era of placing blush over the cheekbones and focusing more on the side of the face. While this does indeed help your face look lifted and more 'snatched', it doesn't serve the purpose of adding warmth to the centre of the face, so maybe it's not as 'healthy' looking as a more classic apple-of-the-cheek placement.

FORM

Blush doesn't always come in powder form. I much prefer cream blush and, just like with bronzer, I usually start with a cream blush then set it in place with powder blush. Admittedly, I don't always do this to myself, especially when in a rush, but for clients who need long-wearing, non-moving makeup, it's a winning combination.

Cream blush

Cream blush has evolved significantly in recent years. I remember buying one when I was a teenager. It was like a miniature toothpaste tube and it was a wet, shimmery, pink cream that pretty much disappeared when blended into the skin. I think it's because of this that cream blush hasn't always been that popular.

> *Thanks to developments in formulation and recent dewy skin trends, cream blush is firmly back on the scene, with many makeup brands making them.*

While my preferred textures are creamy and soft, there are cream blushers in much drier textures now too. These drier versions can be excellent for those with oily cheeks who still want to gain that lovely sheer colour wash that you can achieve with cream blush, but without adding unwanted emollients to the skin.

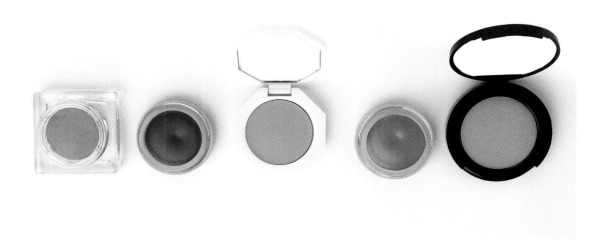

Cream blush can be applied with fingers or a brush.

If you're using a stain (**Benefit's Benetint**, for example), I think it's best to apply it straight to the cheek and blend with your fingers immediately to ensure an even distribution of colour and therefore the most natural glow. If you're not quick enough, you can end up with blobs or stripes, so it's best to work quickly.

When it comes to **cream blush in a pot**, I recommend tapping the flat pads of your two middle fingers into the pot and then tapping your middle fingers onto the back of your hand to gauge how much product you have picked up, just like I would when using a powder.

Next, tap the flat pads of your two fingers onto the apples of the cheeks, then continue to tap in circular motions out towards the top of the cheekbones to evenly distribute the colour.

**CREAM BLUSH
I LIKE:**

– Beauty Pie Supercheek Cream Blush

– Bobbi Brown Pot Rouge

– Sculpted By Aimee Cream Luxe Blush

– Max Factor Miracle Touch Creamy Blush

– Fenty Beauty Cheeks Out Freestyle Cream Blush

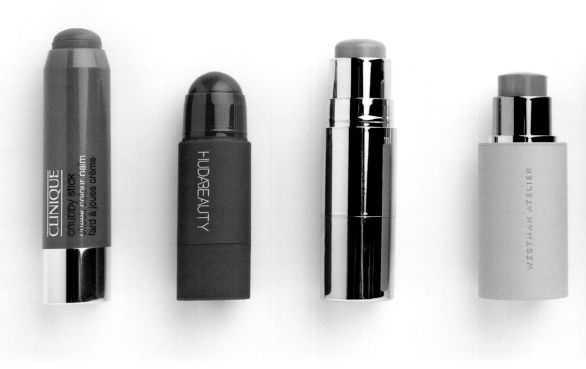

Countless times I have witnessed random people (one of the many joys of London life is people-watching on public transport) dipping the tip of one finger into their cream blush, striping it across the cheek and then furiously blending to try to distribute the intense stripe of pigment. All that's achieved by that is the cheek is dragged unnecessarily, colour rushes to the cheek with the vigorous blending and the blush itself is inadvertently wiped away!

Instead, go easy and try to use the flat of the fingers rather than the tip – you'll get a much more even blend.

If using a brush, then I like the option of a small synthetic fluffy brush (like the **Real Techniques 402**) to lightly diffuse colour across the cheeks and mix the cream into whatever may be on your base.

I really love this technique when using tints too. Tints are a lighter gel formula, often in a squeezable tube, that give a more sheer, usually more dewy finish than cream in a pot.

I will also use a firmer, flatter foundation brush to stipple the colour onto the cheeks.

It's also always useful to have a clean brush to hand. You can use this to blend out the edges of your blush as it can be tricky using the same brush because you could spread colour further than intended, or if you use your foundation brush you could mute the colour.

Powder blush

As much as I adore cream blush, it's not for everyone and powder blush shouldn't be neglected. Textures do vary, but not quite as much as with cream blush.

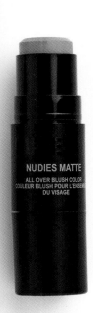

Just like powder shadows, the ingredients and the press of the powder will affect how much colour pay off you get, so you may notice that some powder blush feels very strong in colour on the skin, but you might feel you really need to layer others to build any intensity.

The key difference to powder blush is the finish, with lots being matte, some more satin, some shimmery and some with glitter.

MATTE BLUSH

Like bronzer, it can be helpful to have a matte blush for the days you don't necessarily want a glow (who doesn't want to glow daily, I hear you ask). There may be an occasion where it doesn't feel appropriate for whatever reason. If you have a blemish on your cheek, for example, you don't want to draw attention to it with an illuminating blush formula. Shimmer is notorious for highlighting texture.

Or, if you're concerned about large pores on the front of your cheeks, then a matte blush will be more flattering as the pearlescent particles in a shimmery blush can exacerbate their appearance.

If, like me, there's no such thing as too much glow, then you may prefer a blush with a hint of illumination. Now, using pink highlighter in place of blush won't necessarily work, as highlighters are by nature very light-reflective and you could find yourself with too metallic a finish through the centre of the face. Therefore a blush with illuminating particles is the safer option.

Liquid blush

As well as powders and creams, liquid and gel blushers are a fantastic option for those wanting really sheer, natural-looking colour to their cheeks. They range from super light and watery, like the **Daniel Sandler Watercolour Liquid Blush** or **Nars Liquid Blush**, to gels like the **Iconic London Sheer Blush**, **Glossier Cloud Paint** or **Liquid Lights Liquid Blush** from Sculpted by Aimee. Laura Mercier and Delilah Cosmetics have launched liquid blush recently and I do love the Ciaté Dewy Blush for a bit of glow to the cheek. It's key to note that liquid blush performs best on either naked skin or on light bases like tinted moisturiser and BB cream. They're excellent for no makeup-makeup looks or simple holiday makeup.

POWDER BLUSH I LIKE:

- Bobbi Brown Blush
- Charlotte Tilbury Cheek to Chic
- Rimmel Maxi Blush
- Revolution Blusher Reloaded
- Kylie Cosmetics Pressed Blush Powder
- Dior Backstage Rosy Glow
- Nars Blush

LIQUID BLUSH I LIKE:

- Iconic London Sheer Blush
- Revolution Superdewy Liquid Blush
- Daniel Sandler Watercolor Liquid Cheek Colour
- Rare Beauty Soft Pinch Dewy Liquid Blush
- Glossier Cloud Paint
- Chantecaille Cheek Gelee

Blush hack

If you have a matte blush and a highlighter and don't want to invest in a third blush product, then you can always use a little hack of mine – apply a light dusting of your highlighter to the cheek first, just a little, then blend your matte blush on top and you'll achieve a subtle glow. It works like a dream.

APPLICATION

When applying powder blush, I would always recommend an angled blush brush. I find this helps with placement and to hug the contour of your cheek. Too big a brush and you'll apply colour to too great a surface area. Excess blush or blush too low down can look dated and have an ageing effect, so it's best to keep your brush head on the smaller side. Saying that, too small a brush and you could find yourself applying stripes of pigment. Look for something like **Bobbi Brown Angled Face Brush**.

When applying, swirl your brush over the powder, then tap the head of the blush brush into the palm of your hand. This will ensure the blush pigment is worked into the brush bristles and is stored within the brush, so you don't accidentally apply an intense block of colour to the skin that you'll then struggle to blend, which can happen when the pigment is sitting fresh on the tips of the bristles.

Now start sweeping gently up from the apples of the cheek towards your bronzer. I say gently, as it's always safer and easier to start with a little and add more colour than it is to blend the colour away.

Applying blush to the top of the apples of the cheek is my go-to, but there are other ways that you can apply blush to flatter your face shape.

· For those with **round faces**, round blush on the apples can accentuate the roundness (nothing wrong with a round face, might I add), so apply your blush at more of an angle from the base of the apple of the cheek, under the cheekbones and out towards the temples.

· For those with more of a **square shape**, you may find it more flattering to take your blush straight out from the apple of the cheek towards the centre of the ear, instead of pulling up towards the temple. This can soften an otherwise quite angular (and gorgeous) face shape.

· If your face is **oval or quite long**, make your blush wider across the cheek as you usually have more cheek to work with. If you only apply a bit of blush, you can be left with a lot of cheek without colour, so using a little more can somewhat disguise or minimise the expanse of (your stunning) cheek.

BROWS

BROWS

As someone who started experimenting with makeup in the 90s, I definitely grew up with the belief that eyebrows were bad! Well, not inherently bad, but that heavy brows were bad. All the imagery in magazines were of super-slim, arched brows, almost harking back to the fashion of the 1920s and 30s. I was watching an episode of *Friends* the other day and was so surprised by how thin the actresses' brows were at the time, but really it was classic 90s style. Oh, how times have changed.

In the 90s, when I became brave enough to tweeze my own (it somehow felt a bit naughty – like the first time I shaved my legs . . . ahaha!) I really went to town and got carried away. I became a little addicted to the act of tweezing. Over the course of a few evenings after school I had created what I thought were fabulous, totally en vogue, skinny, almost not-there brows and I was delighted. I mean, my brows made Gwen Stefani's in the 'Don't Speak' video look bushy! I had completely tweezed away the hairs of my brows and was left with a really bizarre shadow from their natural contour. It was a perfect arch of single brow hairs. It was only one day at school when my PE teacher, said 'Hannah! What on earth have you done to your eyebrows?' that I realised I might've gone too far. So mortified was I, that I didn't tweeze them again for a long, long time and thank goodness I didn't – I'm one of the lucky 90s teens whose brows grew back!

You see brows, just like with all makeup, have been very influenced by fashion, trends and styles over the years – from fashion houses to Hollywood stars. Think Marlene Dietrich, who in the 1930s had slim, rounded brows drawn way above her natural brow line. Or icons like Marilyn Monroe in the 1950s who had brows that were much fuller, with her arch often accentuated and at an angle. And then in the very early 60s we had Audrey Hepburn, who sported a fuller, straighter brow in *Breakfast at Tiffany's*. There were more natural brows in the 70s; strong and slightly longer brows in the 80s, then back to super-slim for the 90s. Recently, we have had the most intense brow fashion to date, where we saw brows come to the forefront of makeup trends. Whether perfectly carved out, immaculately filled in, block brows, ombre brows, brows that take hours to perfect brows . . . oh my goodness what a change!

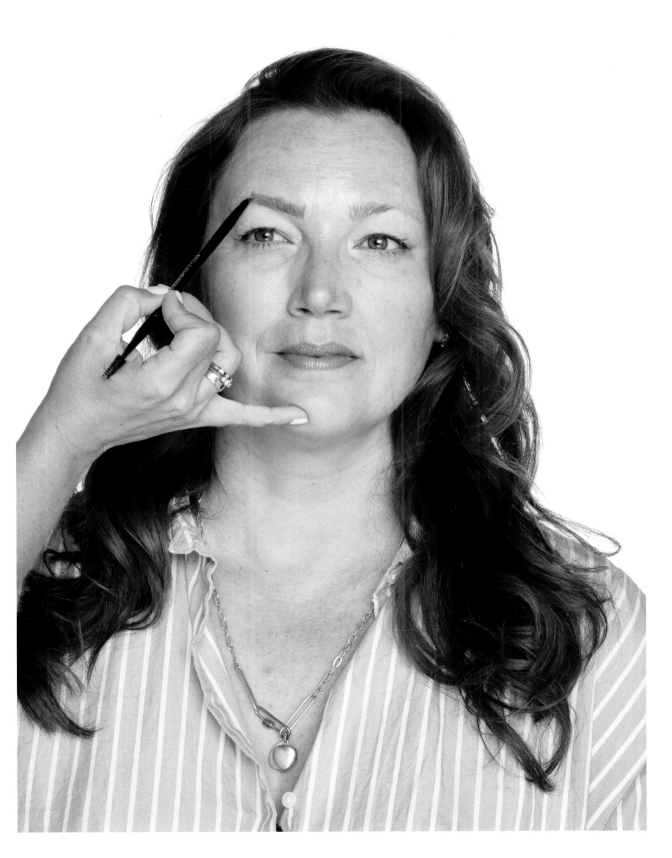

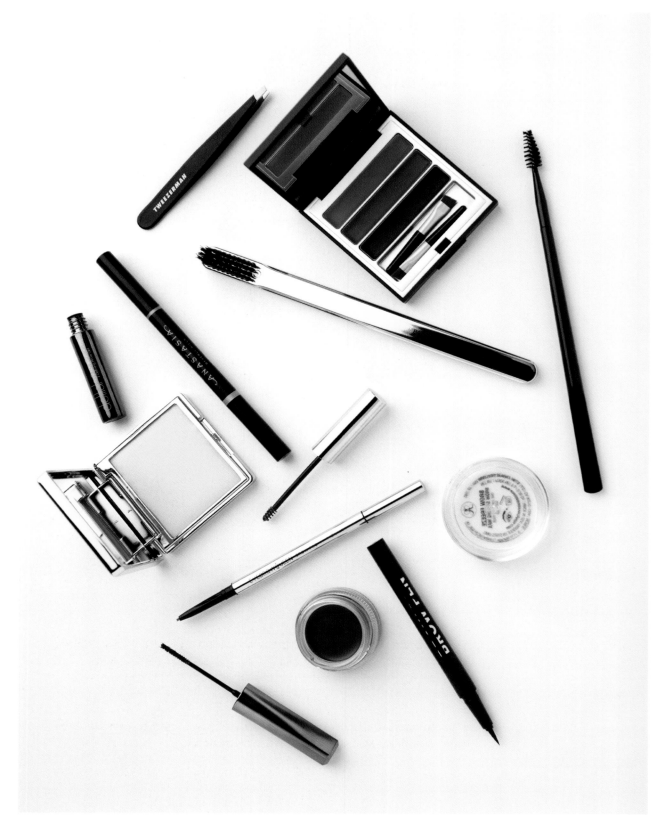

However, thanks to artists like Nikki Wolff, the block brow trend has eased in recent years and we're seeing more love for the fluffy, brushed-up **soap brow** and **brow lamination**.

SOAP BROW

Soap brow is a name given to brow hairs that have been brushed up with the help of clear soap. The soap is spritzed with a setting spray, scrubbed into a spoolie (what MAUs call mascara wands) and then brushed through the brows to act a bit like a glue to hold brows straight and upright.

BROW LAMINATION

This trend started in Russia and is the practice of essentially perming your brows straight so you have this soap brow look without any daily effort. As with all fashions, it's not for everyone, and although I much prefer a spiky brow to a block brow, there are still times when I long to see just a naturally defined, filled-in brow that doesn't necessarily make any kind of major statement. It just does what it is meant to do – naturally frame the eyes and add structure to the face!

How do you shape your brows to best suit your face shape?

There's lots of advice readily available, but if you're really perplexed or are worried about getting it wrong, then I'd recommend you visit a brow specialist to help you create a shape you're happy with, as they are best placed to direct you.

Thankfully, most department stores and beauticians offer brow-shaping services, so a specialist isn't hard to find – just make sure you feel confident with the shaping the specialist suggests before you let them tweeze or thread.

If you are looking to shape your brows yourself at home, then these are some simple rules that I have always worked by:

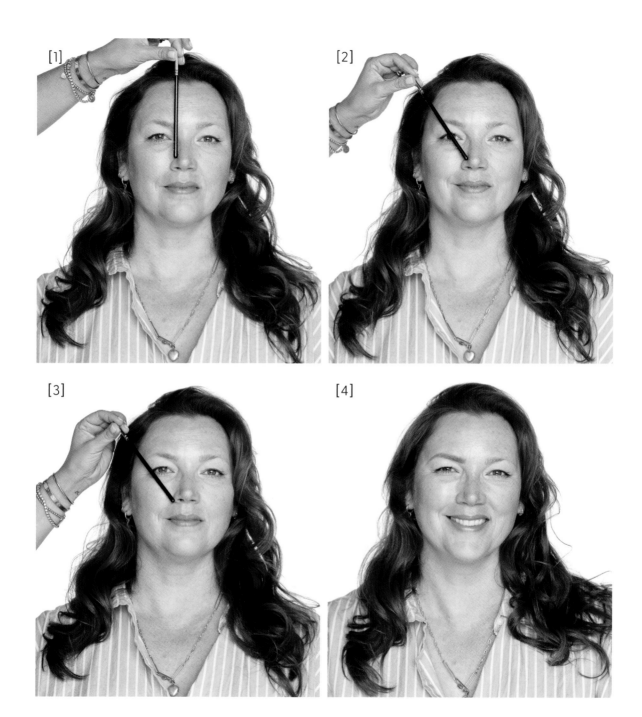

Always start by mapping out your brows so you have a plan, otherwise you could find yourself getting carried away and getting rid of hairs that should have been left in place.

1 I find the simplest way is to use a slim brush handle and hold it from the tip of the nostril straight up. Where the handle lies at the front of the brow, this is where the head of the BROWS START. **Mark this with a bit of brow pencil or shadow**. Anything past this point towards the centre of the brows can be tweezed if you want, but don't tweeze past the handle, or you could make your brows look too short.

2 **Take the handle from the tip of your nostril out at a diagonal to the outer corner of the pupil** when looking straight ahead. This should be where the tip of your **ARCH** is. **Mark it with a brow pencil or shadow.**

3 **Take the brush handle from the tip of the nostril to the outer corner of the eye and lay flat.** This is where the tail of your **BROW SHOULD END.** Again, mark it. Anything past this point you can tweeze but more often than not, I find people have tweezed their brows a bit short so this will highlight where you need to allow hairs to grow back.

4 Once you have the basic three points – where the brows start, arch and end – you can **lightly draw your outline**.

Pencil is usually easier for this, but I start by sketching a straight line from the tip of the brows at the front of the head to the tip of the arch, followed by a second straight line from the base of the brows at the head of the brow to the base of the hairs at the base of the arch.

You can then draw from the tip of the arch and the base of the arch to the base of the tail in an almost inverted triangle, top and bottom, but I don't usually, simply because I don't tend to tweeze a lot from the tail of the brow on my clients as the area is usually sparser than the head.

There are exceptions to the rule, with some wanting to tweeze any stray hairs that may be growing on the temples or outside of the brow line.

PLUCKING ABOVE THE BROW

I've always been reluctant to take hairs from above the brows. I know many that do, but I would always recommend proceeding with caution as you don't want to make your brows look lower than they are naturally. It is widely considered more flattering to raise the eyebrows, if anything, so tweezing strays from below the brow bone is far more effective at achieving that lift.

SPOOLIE WAND

A spoolie wand is so helpful when it comes to brow grooming. You can get them in most pharmacies and beauty departments, but you can always just keep the mascara wand from an old mascara, give it a clean and use that.

I always suggest you start your brow routine by **brushing the brows up**. It helps you check in on the shape, see if there are any areas that need tweezing and it shows up any gaps. It will also prevent you from filling in the brows too low, which you can do if your brows are long and pointing down.

Once your brows have been brushed, I then **use a clear brow gel to hold the brows in place** before I fill in. In truth, it's something I've only been doing for the last few years. I used to always fill in the brows and then set, but my friend and fellow MUA Krystal Dawn taught me this technique and I love it.

Once the gel is set, you can then use your brow products to fill in any gaps. This only works really for those with brow hairs. I'll explain how best to do brows for those without or with minimal hairs shortly.

Brow products

With the rise in popularity of brow grooming there has naturally been a growth in the production of brow products, so it can be a little overwhelming knowing what to use to fill in your brows. Here are what I consider to be the essentials.

POWDER

I'm a huge fan of using powder to fill in brows. Not necessarily brow powder, although I do carry specific brow powder palettes in my kit, but any matte powder shadow that matches your brow colour and hair colour will do.

You should look for a colour that isn't too dissimilar from your natural brow hairs. You can go lighter and should stay away from much darker colours, unless you're fair and your brows can't be seen, otherwise your brows might look more intense than intended.

You're not trying to shade the skin behind the hairs entirely. This is why a shadow colour that is a touch lighter than your brow hair will help you achieve a more natural look, as you'll create more of a shadow and less of a solid block. It also allows for our natural hairs and texture to be seen, which keeps brows looking more dimensional.

Brow gel will also help add texture to your brows with many containing fibres.

When filling in the brows with powder, I find a **firm, slim, angled brush** is best. Anything too soft, and you may find the shadow is dispersed in too great an area. A firm brush will help lay the powder exactly where you want it. I generally use the edge of the tip of the angled brush to then draw the powder through the brows, following the direction of the growth of the hair.

I suggest you start where your brows seem most sparse, so you can start correcting and not filling in areas that don't need it. Annoyingly, the heads of my brows are really very sparse (I believe it's fairly common in those with thyroid issues, though), so I usually start there.

Do the same through the rest of the brow until you feel happy with the intensity of the shade and then look to perfect the edges.

Now, I don't mean draw straight lines at the top and bottom of your brows and fill in (like I suggested when mapping your brows), but it can be helpful if the top or bottom line of your brows is sparse to fill in lightly with shadow to strengthen the appearance of the brows and their shape.

USING TWO SHADES

If you're filling in the top or bottom line of your brows because they're sparse, maybe look to use a slightly lighter shadow shade so this is very subtle. In fact, I'll call out **Anastasia Beverly Hills** brow products here as they are just so good and her brow powder compacts come with two shades – a neutral and a warm – to help with this exactly.

I do find that using two tones helps again to maintain a bit of dimension to the brows. It's absolutely not essential, of course, but if you're passionate about brow grooming, it's a good trick to know.

FIXING 'GAPPY' AREAS

If you have any areas of the brow that, for whatever reason, are 'gappy' or powder doesn't take (quite common with scars), then you may need a more intensely pigmented product (not to be confused with the need for a darker product).

If this is the case, then this is where you can choose between brow pencils, pomades and felt tips. Pencils are the comfort zone for many, but may I suggest you look for a very fine-tipped pencil. They give you so much more control over what you're doing and some are so fine that you can draw really convincing brow-like strokes. I'll often add a little pencil or pomade to a brow once I've done the powder to add a bit of strength to the finished look, but it's not always necessary.

POMADES

Pomades have seen a huge rise in popularity in recent years and for good reason. They can be used softly like powder or very finely with tiny brushes to create natural-looking brow hairs. Most (not all!) come in long-wearing, waterproof formulas and so are excellent for those areas where powder may not take or great for filling in any areas of scarring.

If you're using a pomade, I suggest you take a tiny bit of the product out of the pot, place it on the back of your hand and then replace the lid immediately. This will prevent the product from drying out and also means you can work the product into your brush using the back of your hand.

I tend to brush mine back and forth in order to saturate the brush head in product, but also to flatten the brush head and make the tip as narrow as possible. This will allows me to draw hair-like strokes. I'll then always draw a few strokes on the back of my hand to check that I have enough product on the brush and see how the strokes are looking. It may be that I need a lighter pressure for a slimmer hair look or more pressure for more pigment.

I then draw the brush through the brows in strokes as long as the brow hairs to try to mimic the hairs as much as possible. For the most natural finish, it is best to be fairly quick and confident with the strokes. If you're too slow or overthink it, you can end up with wobbly brow strokes or unnatural placement.

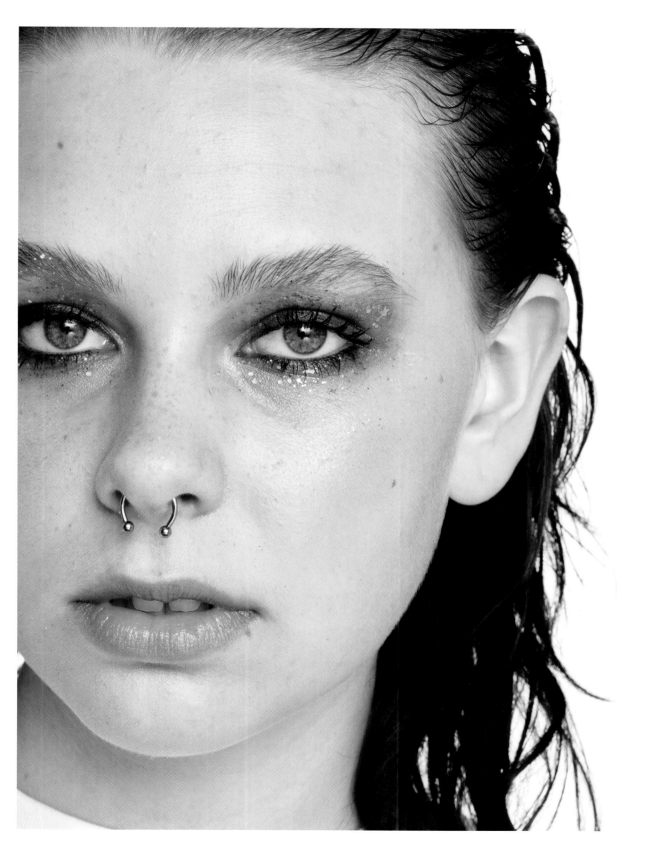

Practice makes perfect

If you're not confident but recognise the need for a bit more pigment through your brows, may I suggest this is something you practise in your spare time while watching TV, for example, or in the bathroom before bed. Practice makes perfect and if you're practising at a time when your makeup isn't important or you are not about to go out, then it really takes the pressure off and, hopefully, it will feel like a helpful exercise and not a chore.

You wouldn't try to teach a child to ride a bike when wanting to transport them to class, for example – it could stress you all out, make you late and create all kinds of negative associations. Instead, you'd take a child to a park when you have some time to practise over and over. You may not get it right first time, but when in life do we ever really do that when learning something new? This is so true of makeup.

I meet and interact with so many people that say, 'Oh, I could never do that. I could never do a winged liner; I could never do a smoky eye,' but how often have they tried, how much have they practised? It's how I trained myself to do winged eyeliner and apply false lashes (which are so much easier to apply on other people, ha!). Yes, I had a few disastrous attempts as a teenager and vowed never to try again, but I persevered in my early 20s and later whilst I was hoping to become a makeup artist. There was a phase where before bed, I'd go into my bathroom with my Boots Natural Collection eyeliner pencil and practise pulling out from the corner of my eye. I did this countless times before I bought a liquid. In error, I bought a very wet liquid liner with a brush tip and had almost zero success. I couldn't get a decent line, let alone a wing, so I gave up until I discovered Bobbi Brown gel liner a few years later, which I found I had way more control over and, finally, I mastered the wing! But it didn't happen for me first time, far from it. My point being, if there's a makeup technique you're struggling with or have struggled with in the past, maybe revisit and try again, you might just surprise yourself.

Back to brows, sorry!

FELT TIPS

I feel I should mention the more felt tip-style brow products here as they can be incredibly useful if you prefer the idea and ease of a simple pen rather than a pot and a brush. You don't have to look much further than Katie Jane Hughes' Instagram page to get the best tutorials in the use of brow pens.

Much like the powder and pomade application suggestions, the idea is that you draw brow-like strokes following the direction of the growth of the hairs to make your brows look that little bit fuller. Another excellent choice if you have sparse brows or scarring.

TINTED BROW GELS

Tinted brow gels are another option that I adore on days where speed is essential. The best ones have very fine spoolies that you brush through the brows to shade and shape in one.

If you don't have many brow hairs, then you can draw backwards, against the direction of the growth of the hairs, and press the wand gently onto the skin to lay some of the product on it, creating that shadow. Finish and tidy by brushing back the other way, following the direction of the growth of the hairs to set the brows in place. Super-speedy and highly effective.

You can get gels that contain little fibres that attach to your natural hairs to build volume, which can be particularly helpful for those who have lost brow hairs or are conscious that they'd like a fuller-looking brow.

GETTING ADVICE

If you're struggling with your brows, I recommend seeking advice from makeup artists in department stores. I always say speak to someone whose makeup, and in this case whose brows, you like, and ask for their suggestions. They are all trained by the brands they work for and can offer you valuable insight, such as really simple brushwork techniques – they might spot that you're holding your brush all wrong, which could in turn affect your application – or they may be able to suggest a colour that suits you better. Do utilise the free help that is available at your local beauty counter.

BROW GEL/FIX I LIKE:

– Soap Brows

– NYX Control Freak Eyebrow Gel

– Charlotte Tilbury Brow Fix

– Anastasia Beverly Hills Clear Brow Gel

– Baebrow G-Lam Clear Brow Gel

– Blink Brow Bar London Clear Brow Gloss

BROW POMADES I LIKE:

– Anastasia Beverly Hills Dipbrow Pomade

– Morphe Brow Cream

– Revolution Brow Pomade

– Benefit Powmade Full Pigment Eyebrow Pomade

– Armani Beauty Eye and Brow Maestro

– NYX Professional Makeup Tame and Frame Brow Pomade

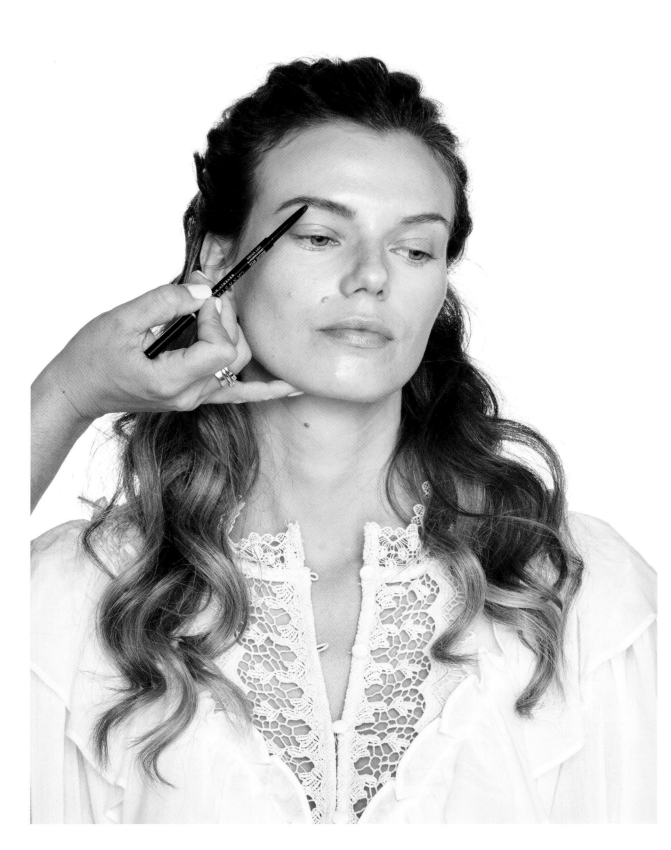

SUPER-FAIR OR NO BROWS

I mentioned earlier that those with super-fair brows are the exception to my rules and can use brow products darker than the shade of the hairs, so let me expand on that.

I actually had the most delightful mother of the bride, Jackie, who won't mind me saying that, as a fair redhead, she doesn't have any brows that you can actually see. They're there but they're very fine and very blonde, so she's never really seen herself with eyebrows.

When conducting the bridal trial, I got to do Jackie's eyebrows and the transformation was incredible! I had to use a colour darker than her brows, so I started by mapping out her brow. I then started to fill in a subtle brow shape with a blonde brow powder – a very light yellowish grey. This flat colour meant I could create what I felt was a light, natural brow. Once I was happy with the shape, I then used a warmer, more cinnamon shade powder that spoke to Jackie's natural red hair, to draw a few hair-like strokes through to create a bit more dimension. I set that in place with gel. So excited was Jackie by her new brows that she renamed our WhatsApp group 'Jackie's Eyebrows'!

I'd also recommend this technique to anyone who has lost their eyebrows, whether it's through alopecia, chemotherapy, trichotillomania or for any other reason. You can get stencils that you use to help you create that first initial powder base if mapping out yourself seems either too difficult or too time-consuming.

> *One last quick point to make is that culture can play a role in dictating brow shape.*

I know I've written about brow mapping and how to find the highest point and the arch, but it must be said that is a fairly Western eyebrow ideal. In China, for example, a straighter brow is thought to be demure and a totally straight, slightly angled brow is considered to be the most attractive.

BROW PENCILS I LIKE:

- Anastasia Beverly Hills Brow Wiz
- Too Faced Superfine Brow Detiler
- Blink Brow Bar Ultra Slim Brow Definer
- Maybelline Ultra Slim Defining Eyebrow Pencil
- NYX Professional Makeup Micro Brow Pencil
- Benefit Precisely, My Brow

TINTED BROW GELS I LIKE:

- Benefit Gimmi Brow
- Huda Beauty BombBrows Full 'n' Fluffy Fiber Gel
- Charlotte Tilbury Legendary Brows
- Blink Brow Bar Tinted Brow Gel
- NYX Professional Tinted Brow Mascara

EYES

EYES

They say that the eyes are the window to the soul, and what fun it is to experiment with shadows and liners, glitter and colour. Eyes are the most exciting playground when it comes to makeup, but a lot of us simply want to know everyday basics that will help us feel polished and put together. Here, I'll endeavour to answer the most commonly asked eye makeup questions. and later I will elaborate on more experimental eye looks.

Eyeshadow and eye makeup looks are as trend-led as any other area of makeup. It still amazes me that while the ancient Egyptians were using pigments as eyeshadows and Elizabeth I experimented with different versions, it wasn't really until the nineteenth century that colour cosmetics became more widely available to buy and socially acceptable for the everyday person to wear. It was actually in the Roaring 20s that the beauty industry blossomed, although the makeup that was made and sold was significantly limited in terms of variety compared with what we're used to today.

So, really, the beauty industry as we know it is only a little over a hundred years old. Shiseido is one of the oldest brands, I believe, having been founded in 1872 first as a pharmacy (the brand's founder, Arinobu Fukuhara, developed a groundbreaking new toothpaste!) which didn't make or sell a skincare item until 1897 (Eudermine – a softening skin lotion being the first product made) and makeup came along even later than that. The trends that we know and love today were only devised in recent history and that fascinates me.

Of course, early eye makeup was quite basic, with rudimental colours available. Navy, black, grey and dark green were extremely popular, unlike the most amazing array of colours, textures and formulas available today.

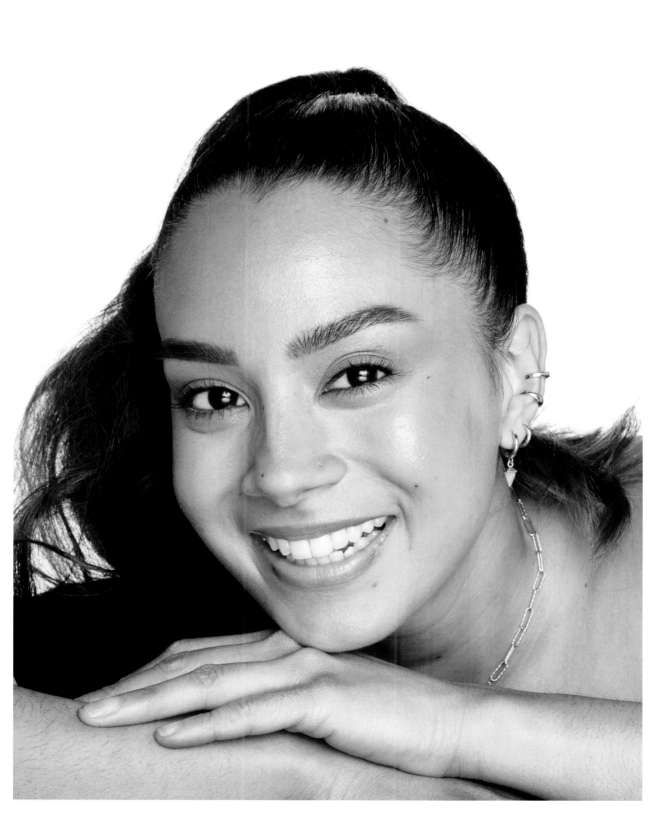

Colour

Can I start by saying again that I'd hate for anyone to be governed by an idea that they had to stick to a bunch of rules when it comes to eye makeup, or any makeup for that matter. Yes, there are guides and suggestions to help, but I hope with every technique or look I suggest you also know that I fully encourage you to wear whatever makes you feel good. It's really important that that's clear. I think for many a few guidelines can help boost their confidence in their choices and decision-making, but it shouldn't be the be-all and end-all – preference and 'joy sparking' are just as important.

COLOUR THEORY

Simple colour theory can be helpful for those unsure of what eyeshadow colour might suit them best. If colour theory is new to you, then don't panic, it's really very simple.

I'll often check my colour wheel when designing makeup looks, but also when trying to figure out home decor shades and fashion choices. It's such a helpful tool!

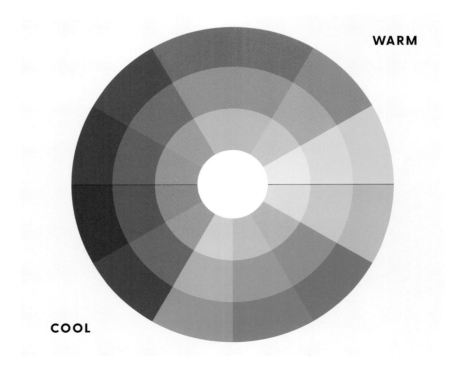

WARM

COOL

Roughly speaking, violet through to yellow are warm colours and yellow/green though to violet are cool colours. The colour wheel shows you which colours are complementary and which are contrasting, giving you an idea of which colours naturally go together.

Any colours opposite each other on the colour wheel are complementary, so can be used to suggest complementary shadow colours.

- Therefore yellow/orange (i.e. anything in the **gold and copper family**) will complement **blue** eyes.

- Colours in the **red** family (i.e. cerise/maroon/reddish-copper) all really complement **green** eyes.

- And **blue** will complement **brown** eyes.

All of which I agree with and I think is a good rule of thumb to follow.

However, I also love a mauve on a green eye, and those with brown eyes can wear absolutely anything, but I particularly love the deep jewel tones as a contrast and to make them pop.

You don't need to wear colour on your eyes daily, far from it, but it hopefully this helps you understand better which colours go well together when you do decide to indulge.

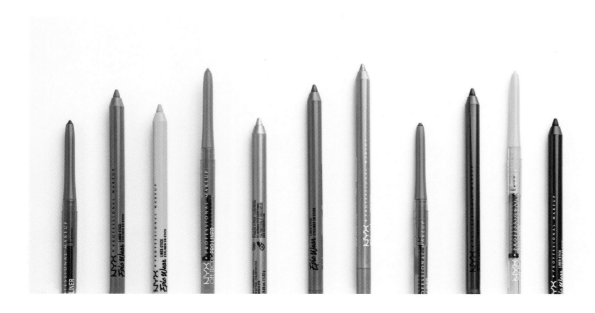

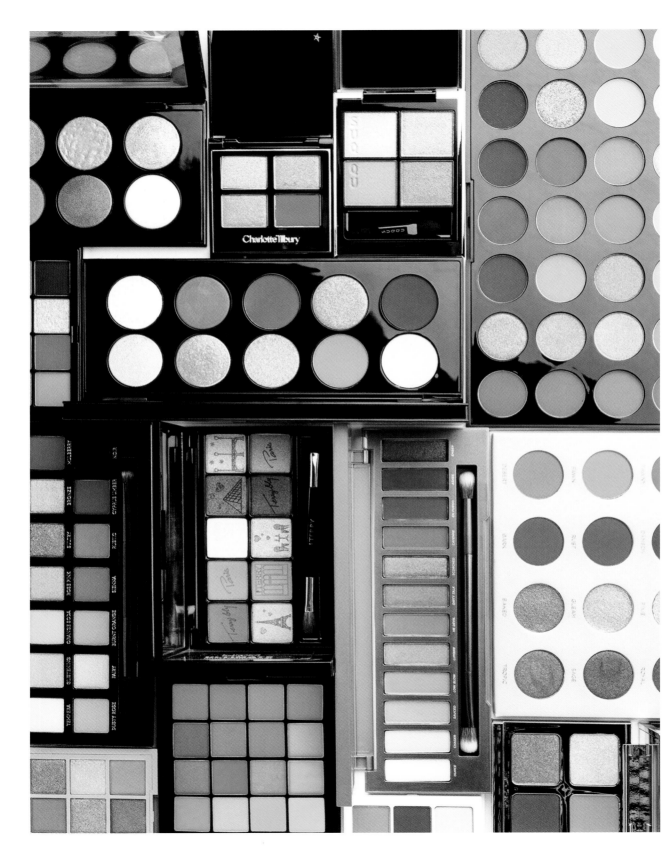

BEST SHADES FOR EVERYONE

I've always been of the opinion that earthy neutrals make for excellent go-to shades for people of all skin tones. It's simply the intensity of the shades that might vary: lighter for fair skin, deeper for black and brown skin. Whilst not the most exciting colours out there, it can be helpful to have a few classic neutrals in your arsenal to help you create simple but polished everyday looks.

My mentor and constant source of inspiration, makeup artist Bobbi Brown, came up with a trio of shadows in the mid-90s that still stand the test of time today – they were called Bone, Taupe and Mahogany. The idea was that this trio worked for just about anyone and Bobbi was right, they did just that.

Whether you're an espresso skin tone, olive, brown or fair, a vanilla-shade shadow under the brow bone highlights, a taupe adds warmth to the crease and mahogany gives definition. On the deepest of brown and black skin tones, I'd swap out the taupe for a black (so Bone, Mahogany and Black) to ensure enough depth of colour. I've always worked by the notion that your liner/definer colour needs to be at least as dark as your natural eye colour, if not darker, to offer the definition you require.

This very basic colour way, paired with mascara, really does work to create simple, wearable, everyday eye looks that are universally flattering.

EYELID PRIMERS I LIKE:

– Urban Decay Primer Potion

– Rare Beauty Always An Optimist Weightless Eye Primer

– Fenty Pro Filt'r Amplifying Eye Primer

– MAC Prep and Prime 24hr Extend Eye Base

– Nars Pro Prime Smudge Proof Eyeshadow Base

Basic makeup days are often when I feel my most attractive, and this style is what I reach for regularly for clients because it's the kind of makeup that simply enhances natural beauty rather than creates that transformation moment.

If you prefer cooler tones, try a vanilla highlighting shade (for black skin, this could be more of a banana or light caramel tone), a mid-grey lid/crease colour and a deep charcoal grey as a liner.

Eye shape

I'll absolutely expand on different looks – I can't write a makeup book and not talk about my favourite smoky eyes – but let's take a moment to talk about eye shape. This is another thing that some people can get stuck on.

> *It saddens me that people can get fixated on what they perceive to be flaws when in truth who declared what 'pretty' should look like?*

I think eyes are a particular sticking point for some. I do understand – I have had times where, as someone with naturally slightly hooded eyes, I've lusted over gorgeous big, open eyes with vast expanses of lid skin and gloriously applied shadow and liner, which I see in campaign images in magazines and on social media. I have to remind myself, like I'm reminding you now, that most of those images have been digitally enhanced and even the model in the image doesn't have eyes quite like that!

Here we will look at the different eye shapes and makeup to flatter each – remembering these are just suggestions and not rules!

DON'T BE FOOLED BY WHAT YOU SEE

Often models have their **temples taped** (think of Jane Fonda's character Grace in *Grace and Frankie* series one, where she shows and removes her tapes). This means clear tape is stuck to the temples and pulled back and tied behind the head to stretch the eyes for more of a 'foxy' eye look. Let's not forget that the image itself can also be photoshopped or filtered, 'stretched' and 'pulled' and enlarged in post-production.

Some of those sporting the 'foxy' eye look have had the increasingly popular **fox eye thread lift procedure**, whereby dissolvable stitches are inserted under the skin to lift the corner of the eye and brow, the 'height' of which is decided by the client, for an eye lift without surgery.

It's hard to explain sometimes to people who produce pictures and ask makeup artists to recreate the look that so much of the imagery they see isn't real, especially when it comes to eye looks.

Quick side note: Next time you feel bad that you can see that pore on your cheek, remember, the person in the picture has pores too, they've just been erased. The perfection is not real it is manufactured – you are real and you are perfect.

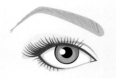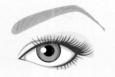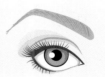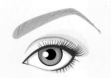

HOODED EYES   **ROUND EYES**

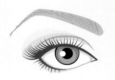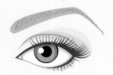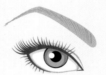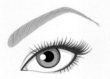

DOWNTURNED EYES   **MONO LIDS**

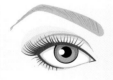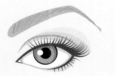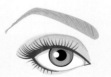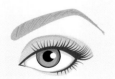

ALMOND EYES   **DEEP-SET EYES**

Tricks of the trade

When looking for makeup inspiration, do try to look for images of people with similar features to yourself. I've spent a lot of time in my career explaining what I can and can't do to recreate images – often because clients will show me a picture they love, but the person in the image has a completely different eye shape, skin tone and bone structure, which means almost no matter what I do as the MUA, I'm never going to achieve the look they so love. The makeup won't make them look like the person in the picture.

I learnt this for myself when I took an album cover of Britney Spears (yes, that's right, I adored her, still do) to my hairdresser and asked for hair 'exactly like that please'. I loved the thick stripes of blond, caramel and brown (this was circa 2002, need I say more) and the hairdresser looked at me and said, 'Oh babe, that's not real, that's all extensions. I could never get your hair to look like that!' I was initially gutted but very quickly I realised my naivety. Of course that wasn't 'real'.

I did, while working in retail, find myself repeatedly explaining the 'perils', as it were, of Photoshop, with people frequently saying, 'No, I want my foundation to look like THIS,' while pointing furiously at a torn-out image from a magazine. 'I can SEE makeup on my skin, I want it to look like THIS,' not realising that the skin they were desperately trying to recreate was digitally corrected and perfected to be completely even and texture free – no lines, no pores, just smooth as silk.

The same is true of eye makeup, with images tweaked beyond recognition and colours enhanced, sparkles added and texture smoothed. Whilst I fully appreciate the beauty of these shots and take great inspiration from them, I do find myself beyond frustrated that these unrealistic, unattainable images can be so misleading to those outside of the beauty industry who, through no fault of their own, know nothing of the tricks of the trade (let's not forget the power of studio lighting, for one), which get images to the point of perfection.

HOODED EYES

I'll start with hooded eyes as this is hands-down one of the questions I'm asked about most – how do I do makeup for my hooded eyes?

> *Height is the key to getting it right when you have hooded eyes.*

If you apply shadow just to the movable part of the lid (the bit below the crease) then the shade won't be seen as it's hidden in the fold of the skin. So it's important to bring any shadow up through the crease of the eye, almost but not right up to the eyebrows. This will ensure you can see the shadow and it also helps to create the illusion of a greater surface area of lid space, thus making the eyes look bigger.

The exact opposite happens if shadow is kept to the lower lid or if eyeliner is too thick – these can make the eyes look smaller and exacerbate the skin above the crease.

JENNIFER LAWRENCE

I always say that Jennifer Lawrence is a great example of someone with a hooded eye. I use her as an example because she is stunning and all too often people think their hooded eyes aren't attractive. Er, wrong! I suggest that those with hooded eyes google her makeup looks. I'm a visual learner so while words are good, I need pictures to really show me what can be achieved. She looks fantastic whether she's wearing makeup or not, but when her shadow is taken above the crease of the eye it is incredible.

So, **take your shadow high up through the crease of the eye**. I like to leave a slim gap below the brow bone (but for a fashion or beauty shoot I *love* to take shadow right through and into the brows). Leave some space in the inner corner of the eyes for a lighter shadow if you wish to brighten the eyes a little.

When it comes to blending the shadow through the crease of the eye, a great tip for those with hooded eyes is that instead of blending with a 'windscreen wiper' motion, pull the shadow straight out from the highest point at the centre of the eye, towards the end of the eyebrow. This will stop you from bringing your eyeshadow too low past the outer corner of the eye, which can make a hooded eye look downturned and heavy. It's best to take the shadow colour straight out and keep the skin below the outer corner of the eye clear of shadow, which will help create more of a lifted look.

In terms of the brows, be careful not to extend the brows too much at the tail end. If the brow is longer than it should be on a hooded eye, again, you could be making the lid look heavy or closed at the outer end. If anything, those with hooded eyes need to ensure their brows aren't too heavy, especially at the base, so they aren't too overbearing or cumbersome. A lighter, fluffier brow can help to open up the look of a hooded eye. If in doubt, you can use the same technique discussed when mapping brows:

Hold the handle of a slim shadow brush from the corner of your nose to the outer corner of the eye to see where the brow should end – for a hooded eye, avoid any shadow on the area below the brush handle.

Hooded eyes or deep-set eyes may struggle to facilitate certain styles of eyeliner, so when it comes to **liner**, I suggest keeping it slim so that you don't disguise or hide the lid and try keeping it to the outer half of the eye. If you take it right into the tear duct, you make the eyes look smaller – we want to keep the inner corner light and bright. Be sure to pull the liner up slightly at the outer corner of the eye. It doesn't have to be a winged liner necessarily, but the act of pulling it up rather than out or, God forbid, down, is that, again, you're taking steps to make the eye look more lifted and open. Just follow the trajectory of the brush handle – out from the corner of the eye and towards the end of the brow. But do not take it as far as the tip of the brow. That would be one long wing!

Those with hooded eyes can line their lower lash line if they so wish, but I will say that I think it looks better if lined with a soft, diffused liner rather than a hard line, which can look a bit blunt. I usually use a shadow or buffed pencil to gently line the lower lash line. Even a light taupe (I often use bronzer, as some of you will know) will create a bit of extra definition. The liner doesn't need to be too strong in tone but a soft, neutral tone liner will help to frame the eye without being overbearing or making the eye look smaller. I do make a point, though, of making sure the liner isn't too slim. One might think a little bit of liner means skinny liner, but a thicker, well-blended lower lash liner actually looks much softer than a thin line.

ROUND EYES

For those with round eyes, I usually focus the definition to the outer corner of the eyes. This will accentuate the corner and therefore create more of an almond shape.

When lining the eyes, I'd start the **liner** in the outer third of the eye, just past the outside of the iris when looking forward, and extend the liner a little – not necessarily a wing, but a small elevated extension from the corner of the eye. By elevated, I mean following the trajectory of the lower lash line. This is a good tip, because if you follow the top lash line past the outer corner of the eye, you may make the eyes appear a little downturned and therefore rounder. This is also true if you start your liner in the centre of the eye, as you'll be highlighting the eye at its highest point and therefore its round circumference.

SOPHIA LOREN

A little extension of the lower lash liner can be beneficial to those with round eyes as it will essentially slim out and extend the outer corner. Someone who did this with aplomb is Sophia Loren. Now, I'm not suggesting going to such extreme lengths – her trick of lining way past the outer corner of the eye, filling it in with white liner and fixing false lashes past the end of her own lashes did the most excellent job of making her eyes look like perfect almond shapes – but the theory is the same. She also epitomised, for me at least, the use of white liner in the inner waterline – a trick for those wanting to make their eyes look bigger (by creating the illusion of more whites of their eyes) or simply wanting to reduce redness.

I'm a huge fan of the Charlotte Tilbury liner as it's more of a peach and not so stark white.

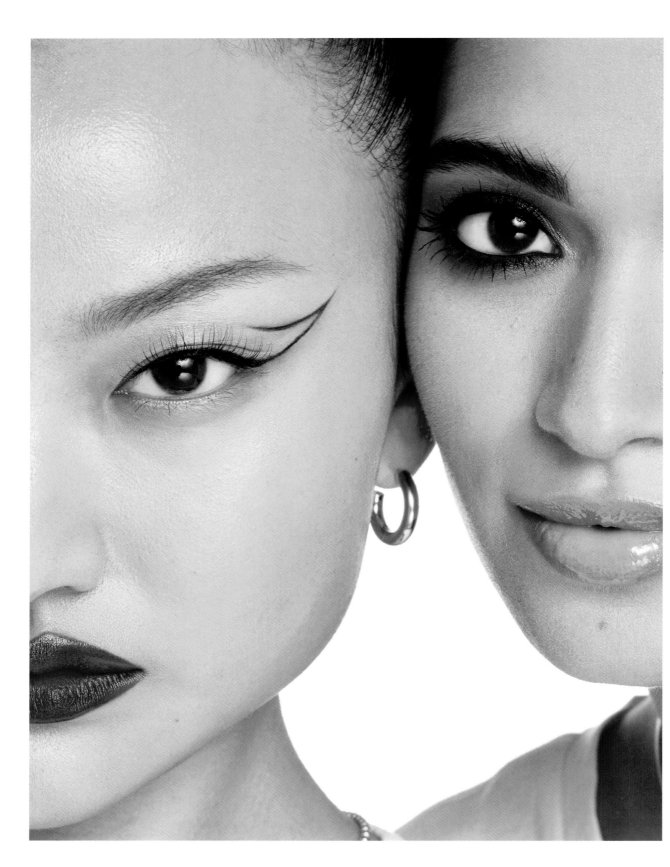

DOWNTURNED EYES

Those with downturned eyes need to be careful when it comes to eyeshadow and eye liner covering the fullest extent of the lash line and past the outer corner of the eye. If this happens, you may be following the downwards trajectory and accentuating the downturned appearance.

> *A trick I learnt many years ago is to stop liner just short of the outer corner of the eye and pull the liner straight out a little from this point.*

If you try to counter-balance the downturn with a flick that loops up, then you will make what looks more like the handle of a ladle, so try pulling straight out to create that bit of lift in the outer corner.

MONO LIDS

Mono lids can quite often be a little downturned too, so this is a liner technique that can come in useful. When creating makeup looks on mono lids, I focus the most intense colour at the lash line and on pulling the shadow up in the centre towards the brow bone rather than accentuating the outer corner, which I might do on a double lid that naturally has a crease.

Whilst some might try to create the illusion of a crease or even use eyelid tape to create a crease, pulling a shadow colour up a mono lid can make the eye look much bigger.

I also recommend **tight lining** the lash line for those with mono lids to eliminate any pinky flesh showing between the lashes. This is true, of course, for any eye shape where there's pinky skin showing at the root of the lashes.

It's key to check your shadow look when the eyes are open, as often the shadow can disappear. Open the eyes and if needed bring the shadow higher above the lash line, around halfway up the lid between the lash line and the brow bone.

If you're wanting to create a bold liner look on a mono lid, I'd also suggest perfecting the liner with the eyes open, as you'll need to create a much thicker line to see it fully when the eyes are open.

Tight lining:
When you line the eyes in the inner waterline between the lashes to eliminate the appearance of any flesh tones.

151

I line the lower lash line too but, again, in a thicker line than you might imagine. Lashes on the lower lash line are often more than one lash deep, meaning that if you try to apply a slim line you may find lashes either side of the line and, more importantly, it may look a little harsh. I suggest using a soft neutral shadow first on a small fluffy detail brush or an angled shadow brush, then sweep it along the lash line and take it right between the lashes. You can always go back in with a deeper shade right up and into the lashes to emphasise the liner look.

It's also really flattering to create drama with the **lashes**. Curling is key on a mono lid because of the shape of the lash line, which tends to face straight out, so a good curl will help lift the lashes so they can be seen well.

QUICK SIDE NOTE

One time I was working with a model in New York with a mono lid and she took my lash curlers from me and curled them herself. Her technique was something I'd never seen before and to this day I'm not exactly sure how she did it, but I can best liken it to when you curl ribbon when wrapping a present. She didn't 'clamp and hold' as you might expect, she closed the curler over her lashes, but not firmly, as she was then able to pull her lashes through the curler whilst still maintaining some pressure. The finish was extraordinary. I'd say it looked more like the curl you get with LVL (a lash lift where your lashes are set in place with a perming agent) rather that the 'crease' you get with a curler. I have it on video and still watch it back from time to time in amazement. It blew my mind. Safe to say I've not tried to use this technique on anyone as I'd worry about pulling their lashes out!

ALMOND EYES

A lot of the imagery we see in mainstream media, at least in recent years, has focused on this eye shape. I wonder why? Who ordained that almond eyes were the most aesthetically pleasing? Someone probably did an equation and decided that it's 'pretty'. Thankfully the beauty and fashion industries are much more inclusive these days, and all eye shapes are starting to be represented.

Almond eye shapes can usually have fun experimenting with liner looks.

Smokey liner, winged eyeliner and graphic liner all work as the almond shape lends itself to visible creases and often an 'openness' at the outer corner of the eye to the brow bone. Almond-shape eyes can pretty much carry any eye makeup look, but my preference is for liner along the entire lash line to enhance the natural shape with a little highlight in the inner corner.

DEEP-SET EYES

Deep-set eyes are often treated similarly to hooded eyes but there's one key point of difference and that's with shading the crease of the eye. Whilst I often do add a shade to the crease on a hooded eye (but straight out towards the brow, remember), I usually don't with a deep-set eye as they can already incur a shadow here thanks to that natural shade of the brow bone. Adding any darker shadow to the crease, whilst not categorically wrong, will emphasise the deep-set appearance and cause the eye to potentially recede even more.

If you want to avoid or minimise the appearance of deep-set eyes, then I'd suggest sticking to lighter, shimmering shadows, the same colour as your skin tone or even a little lighter, to bounce and reflect the light, bringing the eyes forward, not setting them further back. That doesn't mean that you can't wear a dark eyeliner, you absolutely can, but I think it's more flattering to keep the lid colour itself light and shimmery.

TUBING MASCARAS

I know that some with deep-set eyes struggle with mascara smudging on the brow bone and below the lower lash line. This can be due to the lashes touching the skin around the eyes, so I always recommend the use of tubing mascaras to those struggling with smudging. Instead of layering pigment over the lashes, the formula wraps them in microfibres, creating a tube around the lashes that will slide off when rubbed gently with warm water. Sounds odd, doesn't it, but tubing mascaras really work! They don't have quite the same texture as non-tubing mascaras, but the slightly different finish and texture are well worth the lack of smudging.

Mascara

This is my desert island item! Even if I'm not wearing a scrap of makeup, a little mascara can go a long way to making me feel a bit brighter. I think it's because it opens the eyes and instantly makes you look more awake and somewhat presentable.

Mascara has evolved with the advances in cosmetic science, but the first traces of mascara date back to 3000 BC in ancient Egypt where people would mix beef fat, soot and antimony powder to make a paste. The earliest Maybelline mascara, circa 1017, was a similar paste made with petroleum jelly and coal dust that then developed into a soap-like texture with added waxes that one dipped their mascara wand into. Nowadays, with hundreds or brands and formulas to choose from, finding your perfect mascara can be a lifetime's work! It's probably the makeup item I buy most if I'm honest, as I am on the perpetual hunt for the mascara that does it all!

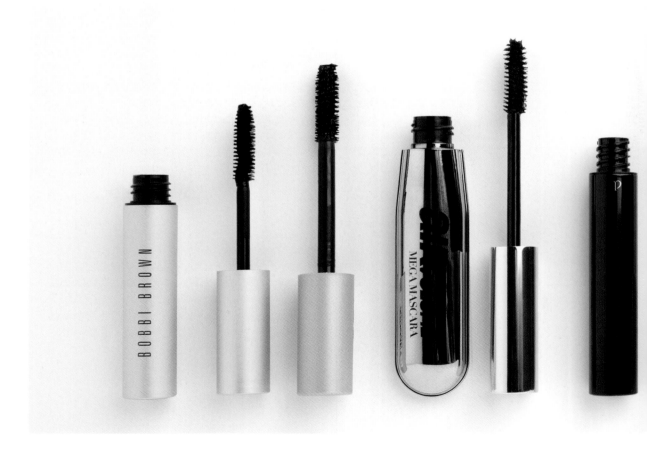

COLOUR

Like all makeup, mascara is a fun way to play with colour. Black is the most commonly available shade, but you can also get browns, blues, greens, plums and pinks. I've always reached for black mascara after a MUA told me early on in my career that everyone has a black pupil so framing the eyes in black will make the pupils pop, but I know some prefer the softer finish of a brown. There is a common misconception that after a certain age one should swap from black to brown mascara but I don't agree at all. If you like black, keep wearing black!

CURLING AND TECHNIQUE

Whatever mascara you choose, regardless of the formula or the wand, your application technique will impact the end result. To get the most out

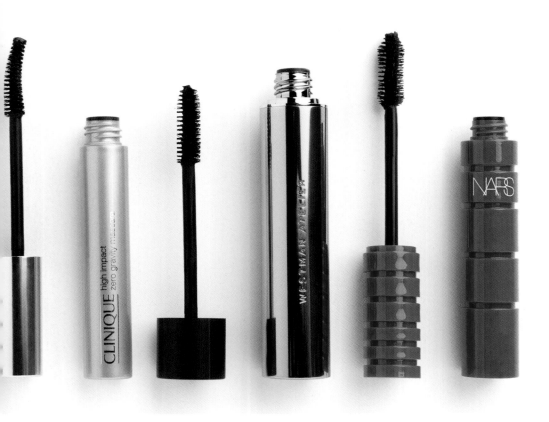

of your mascara, it is imperative you curl your lashes before application. It never ceases to amaze me what gently curling at the root can do to a lash – they suddenly become noticeable.

LVL lash lifts, the process of gently perming lashes, are hugely helpful for those that either don't like curling lashes or can't be bothered to, as each treatment lasts 6–8 weeks. Curling or perming your lashes will ensure more of your lash can be seen from root to tip and any mascara applied doesn't weigh your lashes down. Not all eyelash curlers are equal and there are some that no matter how hard I press or how long I hold my lashes simply don't curl. The curlers I recommend are by Tweezerman, Shiseido, Bobbi Brown and Kevyn Aucoin.

QUICK NOTE HERE TO MUAS

I find it easiest to access my clients' lash line if I ask them to look down just slightly. I ask them to follow my finger until I'm happy I'll have good access to their lashes, then ask them to hold their gaze there. If they're in a high chair and at my eye line this is usually around the tip of my nose. If they're in a normal low seat then the position of their gaze usually needs to be around the base of my chest.

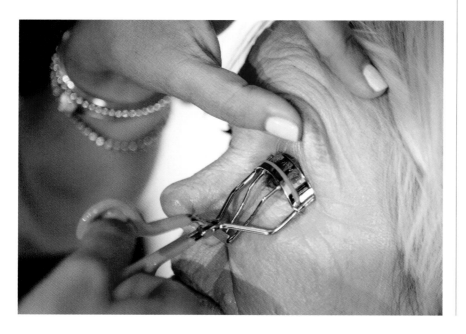

LENGTHENING MASCARAS I LIKE:

– L'Oréal Telescopic Mascara

– Maybelline Lash Sensational Sky High Mascara

– Sculpted by Aimee My Mascara

– By Terry Lash-Expert Twist Brush Mascara

– Chanel Noir Allure

THICKENING MASCARAS I LIKE:

– L'Oréal Air Volume Mega Mascara

– Max Factor 2000 Calorie Mascara

– Nars Climax Extreme Mascara

– Hourglass Caution Extreme Lash Mascara

– Bobbi Brown Smokey Eye Mascara

To curl your lashes

Look straight ahead into a mirror, slide the curlers down your lashes as close to the root as feels comfortable, then very gently squeeze them closed. This first squeeze will indicate if you're too close to the skin. Once you're happy you're not pinching, squeeze the curlers and gently pulse two or three times before releasing and checking the results. The closer to the lash line you get the greater the lift you achieve.

Once you're happy with the curl, it's time to nail the application. I've watched people with fascination over the years applying their makeup on public transport in London. I often see a very rapid application with multiple quick, short strokes of the wand, often pulling out towards the outer corner of the eye. Great for a fanned effect but missing the opportunity to make the most of the inner corner lashes.

My advice is to take your time.

Start by tilting your head back slightly and raising your eyebrows. This will open up the space between your lashes and your eyelid to help prevent getting mascara on the skin. I then gently push the mascara wand horizontally into the centre of the base lash line, slowly blink onto it and pull the wand through the lashes from the root to the tip. I'll repeat this a few times to coat the lashes in mascara and get the most of their length in the centre of my eye. I then repeat the process with the outer lashes, but I pull out towards the end of my brows. I then do the same with the inner corner lashes, but pull with each stroke towards the head of my brow. This technique will help you create that bright eyes, fanned effect. I like to apply mascara to lower lashes too. I find it easiest to turn the wand vertically and use the tip to coat the lower lashes. I find this gives me more control, is helpful for combing and separating the lower lashes and prevents transferring mascara to the skin beneath.

Different formulas of mascara will help create differing lash effects.

TUBING MASCARAS I LIKE:

- Trish McEvoy High Volume Tubular Mascara

- Victoria Beckham Future Lash Mascara

- Hourglass Unlocked Instant Extensions Mascara

- Blink Brow Bar Iconic Tubing Mascara

- No7 Stay Perfect Mascara

WATERPROOF MASCARAS I LIKE:

- Bobbi Brown No Smudge Mascara

- Lancôme Hypnôse Waterproof Mascara

- Beauty Pie The Perfect Waterproof Mascara

- Clinique Lash Power Mascara

- Max Factor Divine Lashes Mascara

Eyeshadow

APPLICATION

Eyeshadows come in varying textures and formulas. From powders to liquids to whips and creams, all of which vary in quality and staying power.

When it comes to **powder shadows** it amazes me how the feel and 'pay off' can vary from brand to brand. There are lots of factors that contribute to how a powder shadow feels and performs – from the ingredients to the quality of the pigments, the pigment weight to the shape of the pan it's pressed into, indeed how 'pressed' the shadow is. I know – who knew there were so many factors at play!

> *A poor-quality powder shadow will be frustrating to work with as you can struggle to get any colour pay off on the skin.*

This is the term us MUAs use to describe how effectively the colour you see in the pan (and by pan we mean the tiny stainless-steel holder the shadow is pressed into) translates onto the skin. In contrast, great-quality (and unfortunately usually more expensive) shadows are identified by their ability to look exactly as they do in the pan on the skin.

The use of a base or eyeshadow primer can really help improve the colour pay off as it can help the pigments adhere more effectively to the lid. The primer I use most is Primer Potion from Urban Decay but you can also use a light layer of concealer or cream shadow as a base.

Classic matte shadows are an excellent makeup bag staple suitable for all skin types and ages. Think of a matte neutral shadow in your makeup bag like a plain white shirt would be to your wardrobe. Classic and wearable, it goes with anything. I'm also an avid user of soft satin-finish shadows, and shimmer and metallics as well as glitter. Yes, glitter! It's not for everyone or necessarily for every day but I don't abide by the rule that those over a certain age should avoid shimmer or glitter. If you are concerned about how a glitter or shimmer will make your skin look then opt for the more delicate, finely milled (i.e. small) glitter that will sit more flatteringly on the skin and won't highlight any fine lines.

FAVOURITE EYESHADOW PALETTES:

Neutral:

– Charlotte Tilbury Desert Haze & Super Nudes

– Too Faced Born This Way The Natural Nudes

– By Mario Master Mattes

– Vieve The Essential Eyeshadow Palette

– Rimmel Magnif'eyes Blush Edition

– Urban Decay Naked Reloaded

– Huda Beauty Nude Obsessions

Colour:

– Pat McGrath Labs Mothership Palettes

– Charlotte Tilbury Luxury Eye Palettes

– NYX Professional Makeup Ultimate Shadow Palette

– Beauty Bay Bright 42 Colour Palette

– Norvina Pro Palette Volume 6

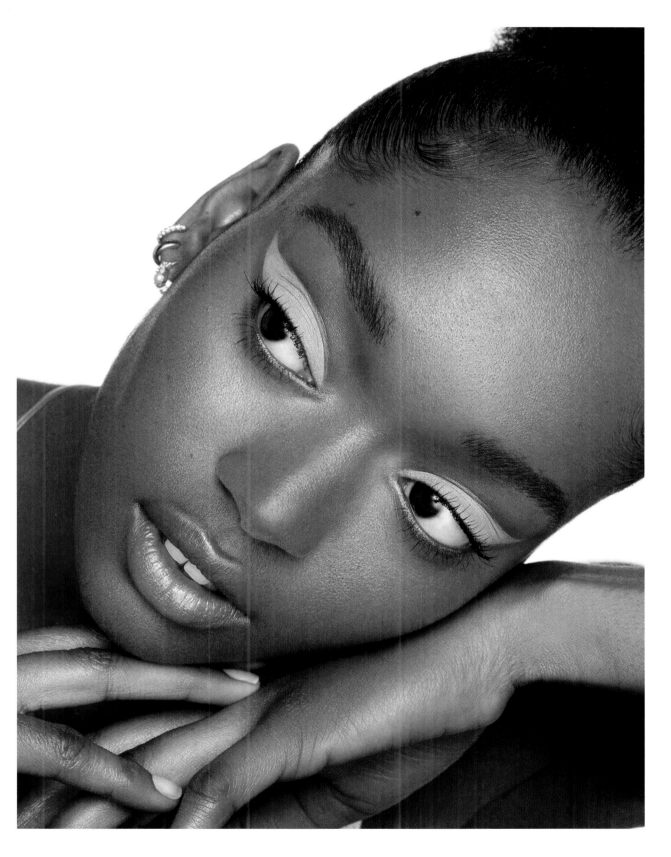

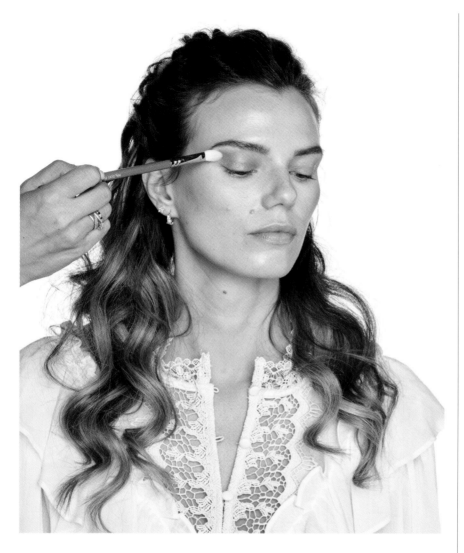

CREAM SHADOWS
I LIKE:

– e.l.f. No Budge
  Cream Eyeshadow

– Bobbi Brown
  Long-Wear Cream
  Shadow

– Charlotte Tilbury
  Eyes To Mesmerise
  Cream Shadow

– MAC Pro Longwear
  Paint Pot

– Maybelline Cream
  Color Tattoo

– Trinny London
  Eye2Eye Cream
  Shadow

LONG-WEAR
CREAM SHADOW
STICKS:

– Bobbi Brown
  Long Wear Cream
  Shadow Stick

– Beauty Pie
  Wondercolour
  Longwear Cream
  Shadow Stick

– Laura Mercier
  Caviar Sticks

– Charlotte Tilbury
  Colour Chameleon
  Eyeshadow Pencil

– e.l.f. No Budge
  Shadow Stick

I use **cream shadows** as a base for powder shadow as it gives me confidence that the makeup isn't going to move. You can apply straight to the eyelid and then blend with your finger or brush. Some might prefer to scrub the cream shadow over the back of the hand or onto a palette and then buff into the lid with a fluffy shadow brush, something like a MAC 217. The cream shadow will smooth the appearance of the skin and provide something for other shadows to adhere to. However, too much cream shadow can start to crease in some cases. This is especially true with metallic-finish cream shadows, so my advice is: less is more. Once a fine layer has been applied you can either leave as is or layer your powder shadow on top.

I've always preferred to apply **powder shadows** using a brush, except for shimmer or metallic powders which I'll apply with my ring finger to the centre of the lid. I do this if I'm looking for a bold colour pay off, as a fingertip helps to 'pack on' pigment, unlike a brush which is designed to disperse the pigment, meaning the finish is more sheer. Generally, the firmer the eyeshadow brush, the bolder the shadow application.

> *The fluffier the brush, the lighter the application. That's true of all brushes and all makeup application.*

A **base shadow** can be applied with numerous different brushes, but I advise using a larger eyeshadow brush for speed. The base shadow covers a larger surface area of the lid and you should apply from the lash line to just below the brow bone.

When it comes to applying shadow through the crease of the eye I like a longer, **rounded, fluffy shadow brush** for gently blending colour through the crease. If you're aiming for a cut crease look (where you draw a fine line of shadow or liner through the crease of the eye, usually darker than the shade of shadow on the lower movable part of the lid) you'll need a finer-tipped, firmer brush for precision application.

For shadow application to the movable part of the lid, a standard **eyeshadow brush** is excellent as they are a little smaller, which helps keep the shadow just on the lower part of the lid.

LIQUID SHADOWS I LIKE:

- Huda Beauty Matte & Metal Melted Shadows

- Stila Magnificent Metals Glitter & Glow, Shimmer and Glow, Suede Shade

- R.E.M. Beauty Midnight Shadows Lustrous

- Rare Beauty Stay Vulnerable Liquid Eyeshadow

- e.l.f. Liquid Glitter Metallic Eyeshadow

PALETTES I *ALWAYS* HAVE IN MY KIT

· Anastasia Beverly Hills Soft Glam Eyeshadow Palette

· Anastasia Beverly Hills Modern Renaissance Palette

· Charlotte Tilbury Bella Sofia, Pillow Talk, Exagger-Eyes, The Sophisticate, Golden Goddess

· Dior Backstage Eye Palette Cool Neutrals, Amber Neutrals, Rosewood Neutrals

· TooFaced Peach Sweet Peach Palette

Eyeliner

For powder eyeliner I love a **short-haired, fairly dense brush** to build dark colour along the lash line and into the root of the lashes. These brushes are also excellent for smudging pencil and gel liners for a more smokey liner look.

For gel liner application a **slim, tiny headed synthetic brush** is best so it glides onto the skin smoothly and you can create a fine line. Note: if your brush head is too big you won't get a delicate finish. Applying eyeliner can be a daunting prospect for many but practice makes perfect. It can feel unnatural at first, but (with a bit of perseverance) anyone can master the art of eyeliner application.

> ### QUICK NOTE
>
> I avoid the application of any skincare to the eyelids before makeup application as the moisturisers and oils can cause your shadow to crease. This is therefore best kept for your PM skincare routine.

When lining the lower lash line I usually apply a powder shadow before using a pencil or gel to intensify the look. I find a neutral shadow along the lower lash line looks so much softer than pencils or gels alone. I'll often use my bronzer along the lower lash line and then add the shadow colour from my top lid in the outer corner to help define the eye shape. I find smaller, round-tipped fluffy brushes are brilliant for this.

For finishing touches like shimmer in the inner corner of the eye or delicate highlight under the brow bone, a tiny brush can be helpful. You can use a dome-tipped one or a very slim flat one to give you the precision you need.

SOFT EYELINER PENCILS I LIKE:

- Hildun Beauty Kajal Liners
- Victoria Beckham Satin Kajal Liner
- Max Factor Kohl Liners
- Rimmel London Soft Kohl Kajal Eyeliner Pencil
- Sculpted By Aimee Brighten & Define Eyeliner Duo

LONGWEARING EYELINERS I LIKE:

- Bobbi Brown Long-Wear Eye Pencil
- Urban Decay 24/7 Glide On Eye Pencil
- Stila Stay All Day Smudge Stick Waterproof Eyeliner
- Estée Lauder Double Wear 24H Waterproof Gel Eyeliner
- NYX Professional Makeup Epic Wear Liner Stick
- Chanel Stylo Yeux Waterproof Longwear Eyeliner and Kohl Pencil

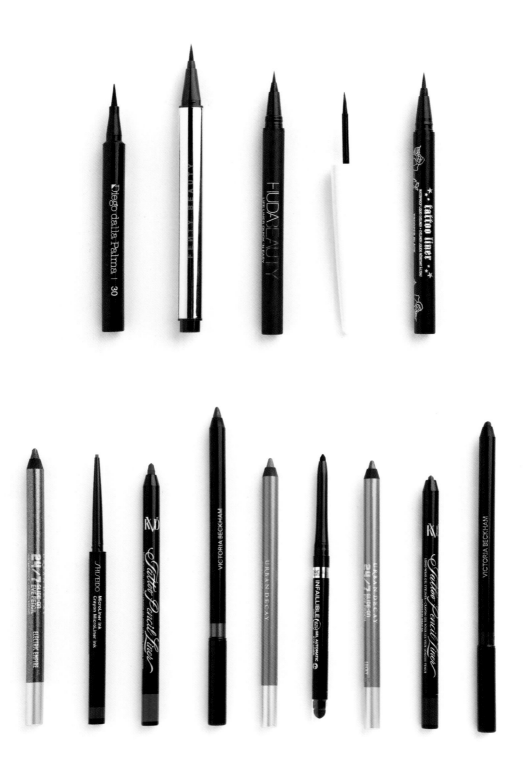

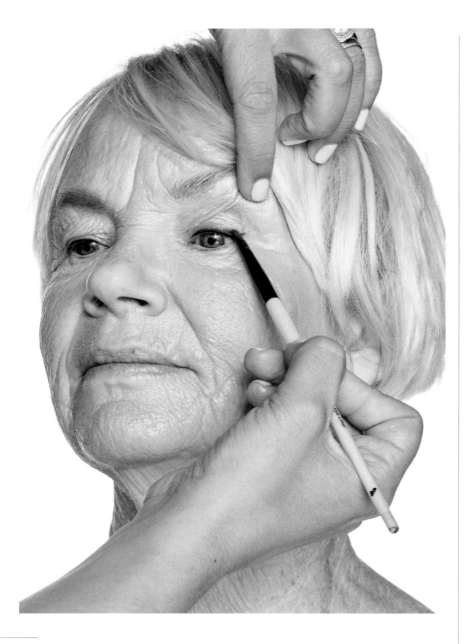

LIQUID LINERS I LIKE:

– Rare Beauty Perfect Strokes Matte Liquid Liner

– Ruby Hammer Precision Liquid Eyeliner

– L'Oréal Perfect Slim Black Liquid Liner

– Benefit Roller Liner

– Beauty Pie Deluxe Precision Liquid Eyeliner

– Stila Stay All Day Liquid Liner

GEL LINER:

– MAC Pro Longwear Fluidline

– Bobbi Brown Perfectly Defined Gel Liner

– Morphe Gel Liner

– Kiko Lasting Gel Eyeliner

– Delilah Gel Line Eye & Brow

– Inglot AMC Eyeliner Gel

APPLICATION

The technique is similar whether you're applying a gel, wet powder, dry powder or pencil and my top application tips for beginners are:

1 **Keep your eyes open.** Trying to apply eyeliner with one eye open, one eye closed can make application tricky. Practise keeping your eyes open.

2 **Hold a mirror under your nose and look down into it.** This will help keep your eyes open and still, keep you focused on the mirror, and, more importantly, you will have a clear view of your lash line. If you try to do your eyeliner by looking directly in front of you it is much harder to see your lash line. If you only have a mirror mounted on the wall, get close to it and tilt your head back. Look down into the mirror and you will have a much clearer view of your lash line and eyelids.

3 **Draw lots of little lines that you can blend.** It's a myth that eyeliner needs to be applied in one clean sweep of a brush. I'll always apply lots of little dashes that I'll then join together.

4 **If you want to create a winged liner, imagine the liner following the trajectory of your lower lash line.** Place your brush into the very outer corner of the eye and pull out – the onus being on out rather than up. A winged liner pulled up too high can look like a curled winged liner. Pulled out from the outer corner will look more feline and elongated.

5 **If you're trying to line a hooded or slightly downturned eye, stop the liner just shy of the outer corner of the eye to avoid exacerbating the eye shape.** Note that on those with hooded eyes you may need to draw over a fold of skin in the outer corner of the eye. If that's the case, just be sure to look down and fill in any gaps in the liner when the skin is gently pulled taut.

6 **Practise before bed, not before a big event or party.** If it goes wrong it doesn't matter, you're about to wash it off anyway. If you practise under pressure, it might put you off trying again!

False lashes

There is a whole world of fun to be had with fake lashes! Admittedly they are not for everyone, but I almost never do a client or bride without them. There are some incredibly delicate, natural-looking lashes available that oh so subtly enhance your lashes to create a slightly fuller lash look. It has the same kind of 'pick me up' power as a blow dry! There are, of course, lashes to the furthest, largest extreme and everything in between.

The biggest barrier I've discovered that prevents people from wearing false lashes is getting them on, so here are some top cheats from me for easy lash application:

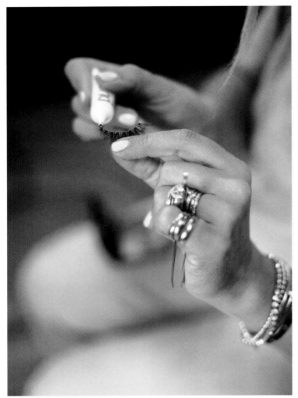
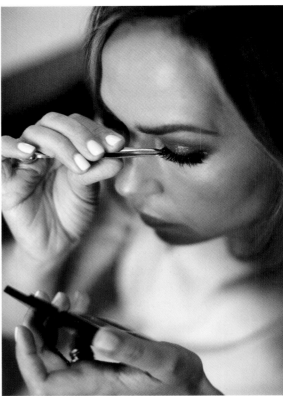

- **Buy ready glued lashes.** Those that come pre-glued just need dropping into place. Simply pull the lashes out of their packaging, hold using a pair of tweezers a few millimetres from the band of the lashes and, whilst looking down into a mirror, place the centre of the fake lashes in the centre of your lash line and release the tweezers. Then using either the tweezers or your fingers, press the outer corner of the lashes to the outer corner of your lash line and press the inner corner of lashes into the inner corner of your eye. My favourites are by Eylure.

- **Buy lash adhesive liner.** This is a liquid liner pen that dries tacky. Similarly, you simply drop your lashes on top of it and gently press into place. I love a black one but you can buy clear ones too. My favourites are **Kiss Glue Liner**, **Duo Line It Lash It** and **Eylure Line and Lash**.

- **Try magnetic lashes.** Some are applied using a magnetic liner, others come in pairs per eye that have tiny magnets at the base – one lash you place under the lashes, the other you place on top and click! The magnets attract and stick to each other with your natural lashes sandwiched in between. So clever!

If you want to try the traditional approach and glue your own lashes all you need is the lashes of your choice, some lash glue and a pair of tweezers. The key is to not use too much glue as you only need a tiny bit. I usually run the lash strip across the tip of the glue or dip the lash band into a small blob of glue on the back of my hand. Just make sure the entire lash band has a bit of glue on it. Let it go tacky and partially air dry, about 30 seconds, before attempting to stick. Hold the lashes in a pair of tweezers and whilst looking down your nose into a mirror, place the centre of the fake lashes into the centre of your lash line. Then gently position the corners of the lashes into place as above.

The shape and length of the lashes is down to personal preference and the look you're trying to achieve, but when applying a strip lash be sure to measure it first. If a lash is too long it can look unnatural and if it sits too far out from the outer corner of the eye it can give the eyes a heavy, slightly downturned appearance. Rest the unglued lash on your lash line and see if it needs trimming. If you like a longer-looking lash, trim from the inner corner or if you prefer a more natural-looking lash, trim from the outer.

LASHES I LIKE:

– Eylure Naturals 020 – the most natural strip lash

– Eylure Naturals 003 – they are ¾ length and slightly fuller in the outer corners

– Eylure Fleur Loves – fluffy ¾ length

– Eylure Fluttery Light 001 – ¾ length

– Eylure Fluttery Light 007 – longer ¾ length

– Ardell Demi Wispies – glam but not OTT

– Ardell Wispies – my favourite full-glam strip lash

– Sweed Signature No Lash-Lash – my favourite individual lash for brides

– Sweed Cluster Flair – my favourite cluster lashes

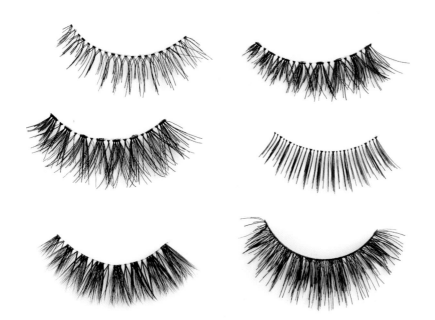

LIPS

LIPS

I love lipstick. When I was at nursery, I loved going to play at one friend's house because she had a little plastic toy lipstick. I was obsessed with it. I used to long to go to her house so I could find it amongst her toys and play with it, pretending in the mirror to put lipstick on.

My daughter was given a wooden makeup set for her first birthday and I experienced similar joy playing with hers! Ha! At six I went on a playdate to my school friend Kirsty's house, and we played with a REAL lipstick – a red one of her mother's – it was the best fun! I applied it and my memory of all the adults being completely amazed that I had applied it myself is so clear. I remember their reaction of surprise and the sense of achievement of having done it so well, perfectly within my lip edge! That's probably where my obsession with lipstick started . . .

Lip care

Before lipstick, a bit of lip care will keep your lips soft and supple and help lipstick look good and last longer.

Lips can benefit hugely from exfoliation, just like any other area of skin. There are brilliant lip scrubs on the market, but I often just make my own at home. Follow this immediately with lip balm to protect and rehydrate.

Lip scrub recipe

In a small bowl, mix half a teaspoon of coconut oil with half a teaspoon of honey and half a teaspoon of sugar. Use this to gently buff over the lips, massaging in circular motions, and this will lift off any dry or dead skin cells while the coconut oil will gently condition. Wipe or rinse off. Your lips will feel soft and smooth. They may be a little red, but don't worry, this is just because you've stimulated the skin and encouraged blood flow and circulation.

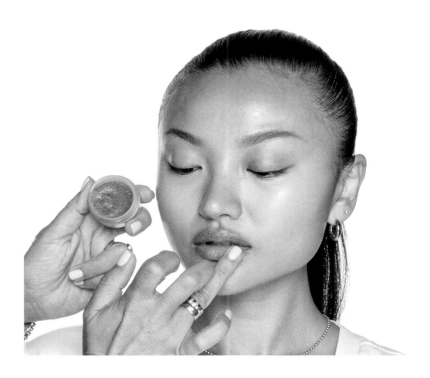

Lip balms

Lip balms vary hugely in their texture but also their efficacy. I've tried many that are light and creamy that feel gentle and relieve symptoms quickly, however the hydration doesn't seem to last and lips don't feel particularly 'protected'. Others are the complete opposite – so 'waxy' that they feel almost dry on the lips BUT they do leave a very protective barrier, which shields the lips from external aggressors. Ideally, you'd look for something in between; just be cautious of anything 'too thin' to 'too thick'.

In terms of makeup application, I always apply lip balm to my clients as a key part of the skincare routine at the start. This will allow the balm to settle and be absorbed into the lips before you apply lip colour. If you apply balm directly before lipstick two things could happen:

· There won't have been enough time for your lips to benefit from the conditioners in the balm, so they may not feel particularly moisturised.
· And more importantly, it could prevent your lipstick from adhering to the lips and will significantly sheer out the pigment.

Apply your balm well in advance of lipstick application and, if necessary, blot off any excess balm to remove excess moisture.

LIP SCRUBS I LIKE:

– Estée Lauder Pure Color Envy Smoothing Sugar Scrub

– Revolution Sugar Kiss Lip Scrub

– Burt's Bees Conditioning Lip Scrub

– Dior Addict Lip Sugar Scrub

– MAC Lip Scrubtious

– Charlotte Tilbury Magic Lip Scrub

– Dr Pawpaw Scrub & Nourish

LIP OILS I LIKE:

– Dior Addict Lip Glow Oil

– Vieve Lip Dew

– Clarins Lip Oil

– Beauty Pie Wondergloss Collagen Lip Oil

– Nivea Lip Oil

For lip balm recommendations see page 28.

Colour

Choosing a lipstick can be extremely challenging – for both consumers and the makeup artists trying to help!

Anyone who has worked in beauty retail will understand the complete joy that comes with helping someone find a lipstick they feel amazing in, honestly, it's like you've both won the lottery!

The flip side of not being able to find someone their perfect lipstick is a nightmare and can be exhausting for both parties – I think mainly because colours – or our interpretation of colours – can be so different.

When someone says a 'brownish pink' they might be describing something that someone else would interpret as more of a terracotta, for example (and the examples are endless, I assure you). I've spent hours swatching new colours and trying on different shades only for the client to want to purchase a colour the same as the one they've always worn.

Or the person who wants to match the lip colour in a picture but can't accept that sometimes the colours credited in images aren't in fact the colours used (often magazines will 'offer' their cover images to brands who will then 'suggest' shades to recreate the look) or that the colour may be a perfect match, but it won't suit them as their lip tone and skin tone is totally different.

Have you ever loved your friend's lipstick but been disappointed when it simply doesn't look the same on you? This is largely because we all have different-coloured lips, which will affect how the lip colour looks. Some have naturally very red lips, some very pale, some have a hint of blue and others various shades of brown. Imagine drawing a pink felt tip over a white piece of paper. It will look different to pink drawn onto blue paper or green paper.

Some lips are lighter and others are significantly darker. It's also common for people to have varying pigmentation in their lips, especially for those with brown and black skin, where it can be common for the pigment of the lips to be dark around the perimeter with a lighter tone in the middle.

Let's thrash out what this means then when it comes to choosing lip colour.

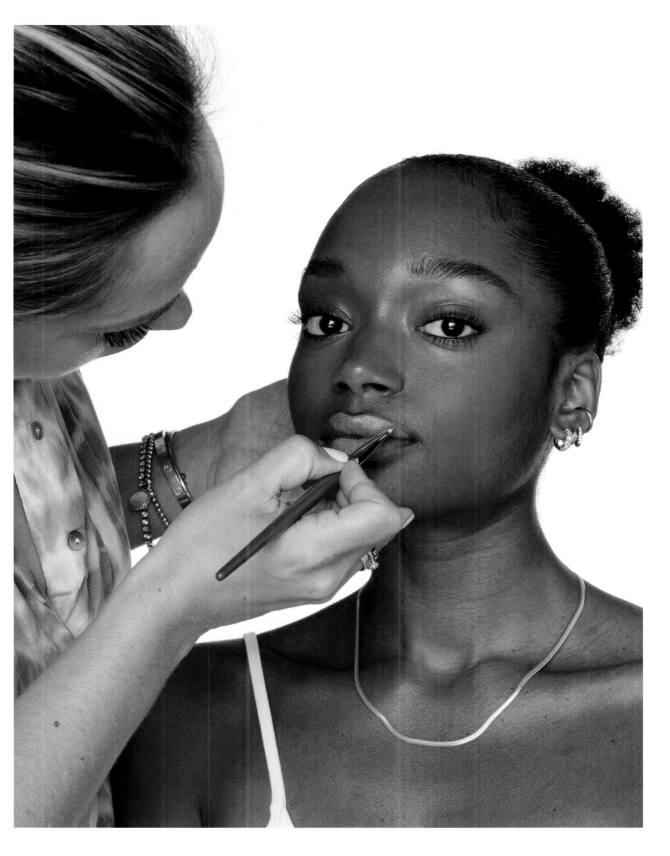

Neutrals

Lots of people love a neutral lipstick, for example MAC's Velvet Teddy, which had a wild surge in popularity after it was favoured by Kylie Jenner a few years ago. However, what suits a light lip tone can look ashy on a deeper lip tone, therefore the tone of the neutral needs to be more intense. That same neutral may look natural on a medium lip tone but then look dark on those with a lighter lip tone.

Simply put, the colour will translate differently on different lip tones, depending on the tone of the skin it's being applied to. And even those with the same skin tone can have a different lip tone, so do bear this in mind too.

For those with differing tones to their lips, it can be that the lighter neutrals still work due to the lip tone being lighter in the centre. It will just need to be paired with a deeper lip pencil that will speak to the deeper skin tone around the lip edge.

> *Essentially: one lip colour will look totally different across different skin tones.*

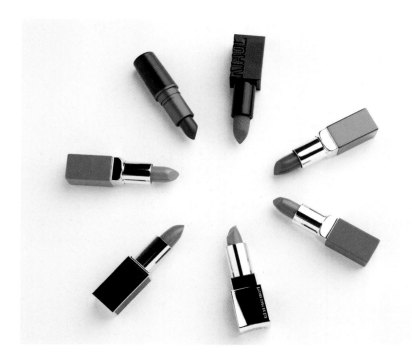

Favourite colours

When it comes to choosing colour, this is far more about personal preference and it's where guidance gets a bit tricky. I say that because ultimately, although many of us want a guide to aid our decision-making, we can all wear whatever colour we wish to.

Yes, some might look better than others, but it's entirely subjective and what makes us feel good might not necessarily be the shade that flatters us most. An example that springs to mind was with the mother of one of my brides. She had worn the same shade of deep plum lipstick all her adult life and whilst she loved it and felt complete and most 'herself' when wearing it, my perception was that the shade was in fact too deep and not what I'd have chosen for her to wear for her daughter's wedding. However, in any other shade this lady didn't feel right, didn't feel comfortable, so despite my opinion, she wore her lipstick because it was her favourite, her comfort zone and made her feel her confident best. She needed that lip colour.

I also think that some people can get stressed and overwhelmed by advice when it comes to choosing lip colour, getting confused by conflicting opinions about cool tones versus warm tones or shades that suit different seasons (never have I been more confused than in the early days being asked to find a lipstick for a 'warm spring', having no knowledge of the 'Colour Me Beautiful' theory) and skin tones.

Therefore, my theory is based on the eye rather than a magic formula. Simply put:

· **If you're fair**, then lighter tones, often cooler, lighter tones, will suit you better – lighter pinks, browns and reds.

· **Deeper skin tones** will suit more intense, potentially warmer pinks, browns and reds.

I'm laughing at how simplistic this sounds, but I think it's a valid benchmark. This is just the place to start. For example, I love the contrast of really fair skin and a dark lip – so sexy – BUT it's a statement and therefore not necessarily what I'd class as an everyday lip colour (that, of course, depends on what you consider 'everyday' – the caveats with makeup are endless . . .).

Taking all these factors into account can help when choosing lip colours but they shouldn't hold you back from colours you simply love.

MY FAVOURITE LIPSTICKS:

Sheer:

– Sisley Phyto-Rouge Shine

– e.l.f. Sheer Slick Lipstick

– Kiko Glossy Dream Sheer Lipstick

– Glossier Ultralip

– Chanel Rouge Coco Flash

– Bobbi Brown Crushed Shine Jelly Stick

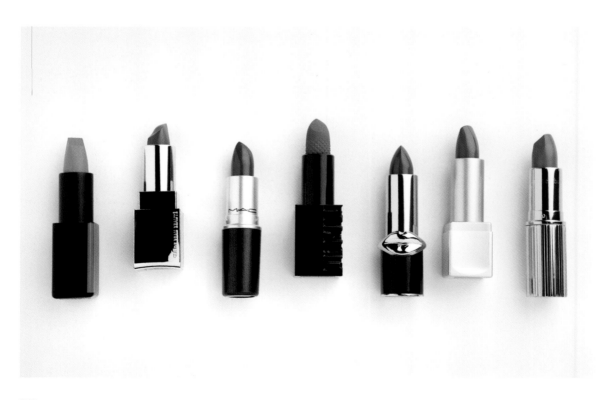

176

Cool and warm undertones

What constitutes a cool tone and what makes for a warm tone can be confusing, so let me try to explain.

Firstly, while I don't think it's the be-all and end-all and shouldn't guide your every makeup decision, it can be helpful to recognise your own skin undertone:

Those with **cool undertones**, generally speaking, look better in silver jewellery. You may also notice that the veins in your hands and wrists look quite blue, which is why the silver tone is more complementary than the gold, which is contrasting and can make you look yellow. It's also true that those with cooler undertones tend to burn easily in the sun and often (but not always) have paler eyes.

Cool colours therefore (thanks again colour wheel, see page 140) are essentially those with blue/green/light purple undertones.

Those with **warmer undertones** generally suit gold better, tan more easily and their veins appear more green than blue.

Warm colours therefore are those in the red/orange/yellow family.

Then those with **neutral undertones** are those that suit both silver and gold, can burn in the sun but then tan, and their veins look both green and blue.

With neutral shades not actually appearing on the colour wheel, neutral colours are essentially black, white, cream, grey and the many differing intensities and hues of tones that make beige.

MY FAVOURITE LIPSTICKS:

Satin finish:

− MAC Satin lipsticks

− Bobbi Brown Luxe Lip Colour

− Lisa Eldridge Luxuriously Lucent Lip Colour

− Hourglass Unlocked Satin Creme Lipsticks

− bareMinerals Mineralist Hydra Smoothing Lipstick

− L'Oréal Color Riche Lipsticks

− Armani Lip Power

Matte:

− Lisa Eldridge True Velvet Lip Colour

− Pat McGrath MatteTrance Lipstick

− MAC Matte Lipstick

− Huda Beauty Power Bullet Matte Lipstick

− Beauty Pie Futurelipstick Matte All Day Long

− Nars Powermatte Lipstick

− Shiseido ModernMatte Powder Lipstick

FINDING LIP COLOURS

Trying on lip colours can be time-consuming, so I like to recommend clients pick up whichever colours immediately catch their eye. There's something intuitive about gut instinct and it plays a huge part in colour selection.

Testing lip colours

Take each lip shade and apply to your fingertips – sounds weird but bear with me – then one by one, take your fingertip up to your mouth and look in the mirror to see how the shade looks against your lips and skin. You can quickly deduce which ones you like and which ones simply don't look right and that you can discount, thus narrowing down the number you wish to try on entirely.

From there, it's a case of personal preference. Which do you like best when you try it on? Which makes you feel pretty?

And remember, a lip colour that suits your skin tone will look good regardless of what you wear. You don't need to match your lipstick to your outfit.

MY FAVOURITE LIPSTICKS:

Liquid:

– Hourglass Velvet Story Lip Cream

– Kylie Jenner Matte Liquid Lipstick

– Kylie Jenner Lip Blush

– Huda Beauty Liquid Matte Lipstick

– Max Factor Lipfinity

– Revolution IRL Whipped Lip Creme

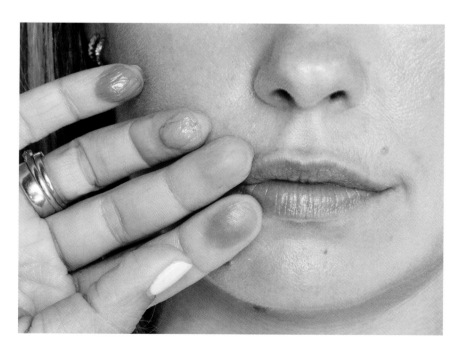

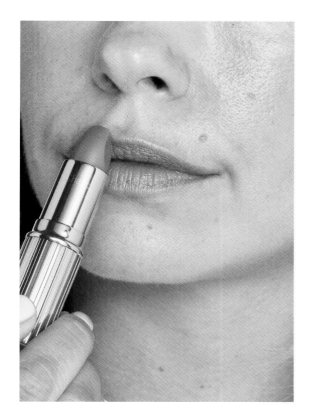
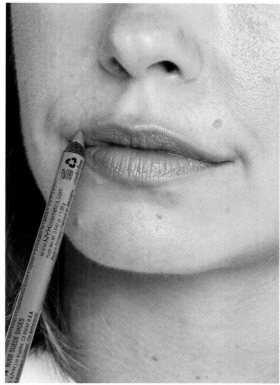

Lip pencil

When it comes to lip pencil, I've always preferred either matching the lip pencil to the shade of your lips to simply tidy your lip edge before lip colour application OR matching the lip pencil to the lip colour you wish to wear. I think this was born from my experience as a 90s teenager, when it was common to see really contrasting lip pencils and lipsticks worn together that, while not wrong per se, didn't look at all natural. Anyone else remember the dark brown lip pencil paired with exceptionally light lipstick? Or the deep cherry paired with frosted pink?

Of course, that's still done today, but I think the more modern way of wearing a multi-tonal lip is to create a softer, ombre look, where the shades are gradually blended so the contrast is still there but significantly less. The exception here, of course, is for those with naturally different tones in their lips – in that the application of the various tones is mimicking the shades naturally present, therefore enhancing and complementing, not creating, something that doesn't already exist.

If you chose to wear a lip pencil the same colour as your lips to tidy your lip edge – maybe because your lip edge is somewhat undefined or uneven, for example – I recommend applying your liner first, so you know within what parameters you'll want to apply your lipstick.

If you are using a lip colour the same shade as your lipstick to perfect the edge of the lipstick, then I apply it after.

If I'm doing a red lip on a client, for example, I'll apply the lip colour as perfectly as possible (I use a brush when working on others but usually just apply straight from the bullet when applying on myself), then use the lip pencil to carefully perfect the edge.

Whether applying to myself or others, I do think it really helps to 'anchor' your hand by holding your little finger against the chin (you often see MUAs doing this with small sponges on their fingers – this is to prevent moving the makeup underneath) to help steady your hand and help you create a smoother finish.

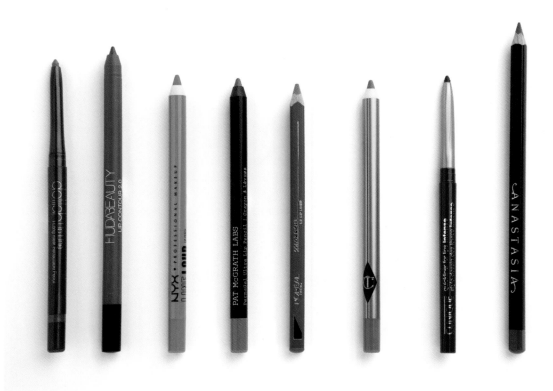

I also keep the pencil in contact with the skin and do little movements, back and forth, rather than trying to draw freehand or lifting the tip of the pencil with each stroke. By keeping the pencil in contact with the skin, you're eliminating the risk of replacing the nib either inside or outside of the trajectory you were last on and are more likely to keep to the line you're aiming for.

Using a lip pencil to change lip shape

Some may be surprised to hear this, but I'm quite a fan of augmenting lip shape with lip pencil. Yes, I usually err on the side of natural when it comes to makeup, but I do love the power of switching up a lip shape with a bit of lip pencil:

· Over-lining slightly to give the lips a fuller appearance.

· Over-lining the outer corner to create a wider-looking lip, something Audrey Hepburn perfected.

· Lining within the outer corner and concealing the exposed bit of lip for a narrower lip.

· Sharpening or softening the cupid's bow.

The options are endless and if done well, look fantastic. The key is to do your shaping subtly. As soon as you overdo it, whether that's overlining too far outside the natural lip edge or making the cupid's bow too tall, that's when it can look more theatrical than natural, but don't be afraid to experiment.

One other tip when it comes to lip pencil is that you can use the pencil to create a stain for your lipstick to adhere to. If you struggle to keep your lipstick on, you may find it helpful to invest in a long-wear lip pencil, which you then apply all over the lip before applying your lipstick. The lip pencil will lock in place, so if your lipstick wears off for whatever reason, you're still left with the shade. I also use this trick if I want to avoid being left with a ring of obvious lip liner around the perimeter of the lips as your lipstick wears off.

LIP PENCILS I LIKE:

– Doll Beauty Lipliners

– Revolution IRL Filter Finish Lip Definer

– Charlotte Tilbury Lip Cheat

– NYX Professional lip liners

– Huda Beauty Lip Contour 2.0

– Kylie Jenner Lip Liner

– Vieve Modern Lip Definer

– Pat McGrath PermaGel Ultra Lip Pencil

– MAC lipliners

– Rare Beauty Kind Words Lip pencils

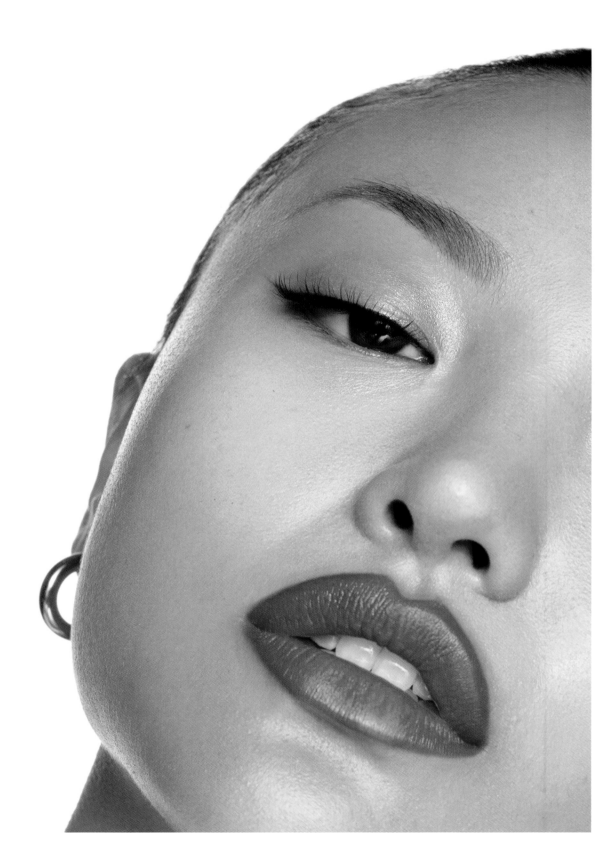

Textures & formulas

Lipsticks vary wildly in texture and formula and therefore wear – from sheer and hydrating, to matte and long-lasting and everything in between!

Sheer balm-based lipsticks are brilliant if you don't like anything too bold or prefer a softer-looking lip colour. They are a great option if you want to try a new colour but aren't ready to commit to a full lipstick. Red lipstick is the perfect example. If you're nervous about wearing such a bold colour, then a sheer lipstick can be a great place to start.

Classic lipsticks are probably what we're most familiar with and are generally more opaque in finish and wear reasonably well. Moisturising or 'satin finish' lipsticks won't last as long due to their more slippery texture. Matte finishes will last longer due to their drier, more pigment-dense formula that adheres better to the lips.

Liquid lipsticks, matte ones in particular, have seen a huge rise in popularity in recent years. American reality TV star and cosmetic brand owner Kylie Jenner became the world's youngest billionaire thanks to her best-selling 'Lip Kits', the first drop of which sold out within minutes of launching. Their matte finish and staying power saw a swathe of brands and influencers rush to make their own and I'm not ashamed to say that I was influenced and bought the Huda Beauty Liquid Lipstick vault at great expense. I also own nearly every shade of the Kylie Cosmetics liquid lipsticks. I use them with my clients as a long-wearing base lip colour then add gloss on top, especially if my client has a long day and no time for touch-ups.

Some of my very favourite lip products are in the more sheer, moisturising family as my preference is for hydrated, shiny-looking lips. I think it makes my lips look fuller, but it's almost impossible to find a moisturising lip product that lasts a long time.

In contrast, it is hard to find a moisturising matte lipstick as too many emollients negate the matte finish.

It can be challenging to find lipsticks that meet all criteria, especially if the criteria are opposing. So, if you like a glossy finish, then a long-wear matte might be best applied underneath for occasions when you know you want long wear.

Similarly, if you want long wear but don't like a matte finish, then a balm or gloss on top can make the long-wear lip product glossier and more comfortable.

GETTING FULLER LIPS

I know some worry that matte lipstick may make thin lips look thinner, but that is not entirely true. Although I admit that it won't make thin lips appear any fuller – that's where the shine of a gloss can help, by bouncing and reflecting the light – you can use highlight and contour to enhance the lip shape for the matte lipstick. Add a little highlighter to the top of the cupid's bow to create the illusion of a full lip edge or 'lip flip', where your lip edge is naturally a bit more pronounced.

Contour can be used to shade around the lip edge to create the illusion of fuller lips. By faking where the lip edge recedes, you can enlarge your lip edge. This can look odd if not done well and blended out, so it's not necessarily something I recommend without a lot of practice. You may have seen this on social media along with all manner of odd hacks for creating fuller-looking lips, such as sucking their lips into tiny pots and pinching their lips between eyelash curlers – crazy practices that I absolutely do not encourage!

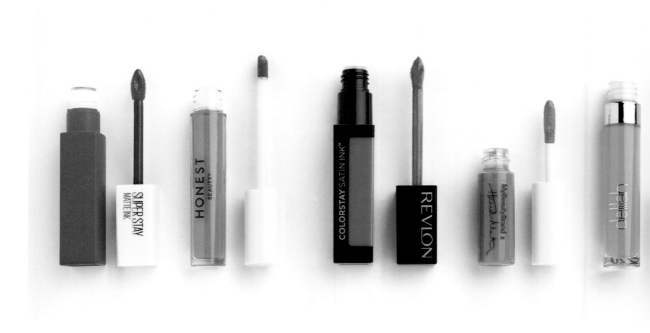

AESTHETIC PROCEDURES

I know that for a lot of people insecurities about thin lips can be all-consuming. Whilst I don't encourage aesthetic procedures as a 'solution', I do know that well-administered dermal filler in the lips can create very natural results that can boost people's confidence. I've had the pleasure of working on the revamped show *10 Years Younger* and have witnessed some truly incredible transformations, not just of appearance but more importantly of confidence, thanks to some TLC from the experts and the sharing of their expertise.

Please don't get me wrong, I'm not promoting or suggesting anyone needs aesthetic procedures. It is of course a very personal choice and something only adults should do if they are completely sure and after professional consultations. I certainly don't advocate young people having extreme procedures. It breaks my heart to see young people with overly filled lips, cheeks and jawlines, but it would be naive to think all aesthetic procedures are bad, because they're not. They should be used with caution and consideration and only ever done by a trained professional.

LIP GLOSSES I LIKE:

– Maybelline Lifter Gloss

– Clarins Lip Perfector

– Fenty Beauty Gloss Bomb

– Kiko 3D Hydra Lipgloss

– Shiseido Gel Gloss

– Chanel Rouge Coco Gloss

Lip gloss

I'm thrilled that lip gloss has made a bit of a comeback.

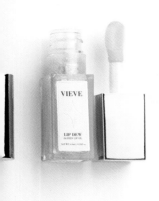

Matte had been the order of the day for a while, a bit of a knee-jerk reaction to the endless gloss of the 90s perhaps (hands up if you used to collect Juicy Tubes too? They were on my Christmas list for many years!). Lip glosses are intended to create shiny, full-looking lips. Worn on top of lipstick or alone, gloss can make lips look plump and hydrated thanks to light bouncing off the sheen. Tinted glosses – Clarins Lip Perfectors are my all-time favourite – are excellent options for days when you don't want to commit to a lipstick but still want a bit of colour and conditioning.

They can be a little sticky, so aren't ideal on a windy day if you have long hair, but a dab of something shiny on the lips can be the perfect finisher. Whether it's a pat of Dr PawPaw balm or sparkly gloss, the light reflection and attention-focusing sheen can help you feel more glamorous.

EXTRAS: HIGHLIGHTER & GLITTER

HIGHLIGHTER

I first encountered highlighter when I was 12 years old, at a sleepover at my friend Miriam's house. One of her other friends had the most incredible glow to her cheeks. I'd never seen anything like it and was absolutely mesmerised. What was this ethereal luminosity?

Once I plucked up the courage to ask, it turned out it was a highlighting pan stick from Max Factor. Well, that was it, I had to have one. It felt expensive to buy at the time, but I treasured it and used it on special occasions. Although the finish was subtle, it made me feel amazing and I was buoyed knowing I had this secret-weapon miracle skin illuminator in my makeup bag.

Sadly, I believe the highlighting stick I originally bought no longer exists but there many alternatives available from numerous brands in lots of different textures and finishes. Powder highlighters are probably the most common, swiftly followed by liquids and creams.

A SUBTLE GLOW

> *One of my favourite ways of using highlighter is to use a liquid one before foundation.*

I apply a liquid highlighter to the higher points of the face – always top of the cheeks but sometimes bridge of the nose and temples too – before the base to create that 'lit from within' glow.

In fact, on the very first episode of the revamped *10 Years Younger*, I used Becca Backlight Priming Filter (it's a travesty that the brand is no more) under the contributor Gail's makeup and, wow – she looked like a film star on the red carpet during her reveal scene – but the cameraman took me to one side and told me that in television you can't use as much highlighter as it's really strong on camera and you will appear shiny. Either way, Gail's big reveal look is still one of my favourites thanks to the incredible glow she had by using a subtle highlighter under her foundation. Charlotte Tilbury's Hollywood Flawless Filter is an excellent choice for this.

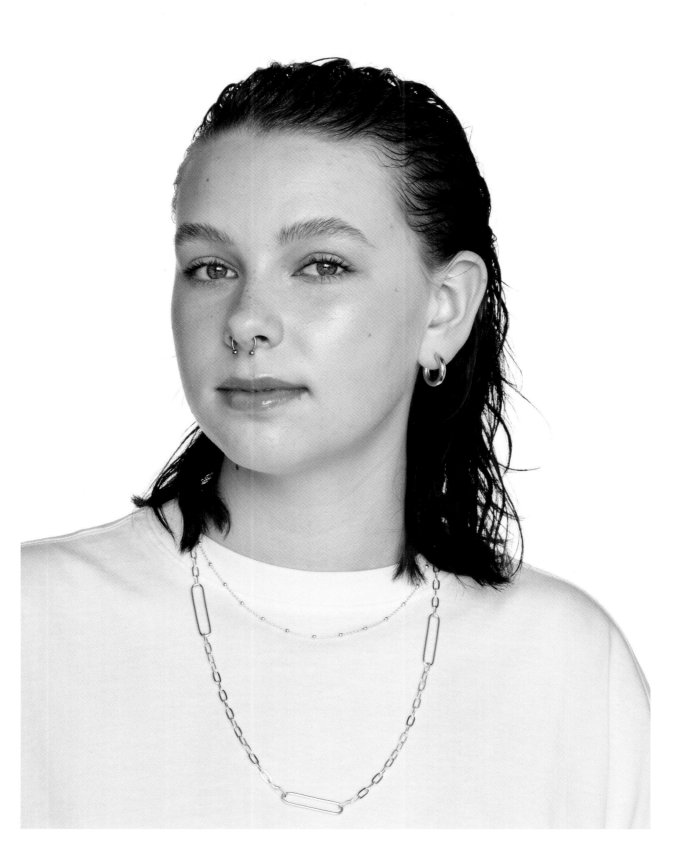

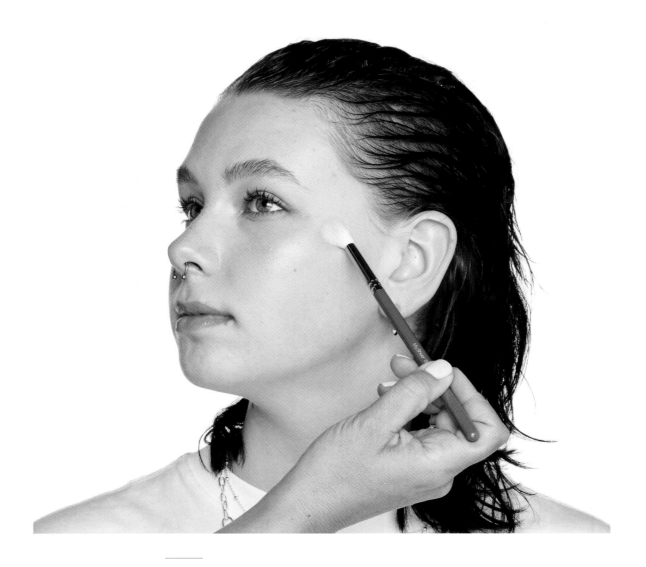

A STRONGER GLOW

For more of a glow, you can mix your foundation with a liquid highlighter. Just be wary that highlighter can emphasise the appearance of pores, so if you're concerned about pore size, then it's probably best to keep your highlighter to just a few areas rather than all over. Also, if you have black or brown skin, look for highlighters that have more golden/red light reflective particles, as those with too much silver can look grey and ashy and cause the opposite of the desired effect, which is to make the skin look brighter and more radiant.

AN INTENSE GLOW

For the most intense glow, apply your highlighter on top of your base makeup. I do love liquid highlighter blended into foundation on the top of the cheeks (either with fingers or a fluffy brush) before any powder product is applied, followed by blush on top. Again, it creates that 'lit from within' glow. You can, of course, use liquid highlighter at the very end of your makeup for a finishing touch, but this works best when it's the last step and over liquid makeup.

It can be tricky to layer liquid highlighter over powdery formulas as it may cause them to split, or you can find yourself wiping away the makeup beneath whilst blending. This doesn't seem to happen when blending cream into cream. I learnt this the hard way one Christmas. I was about 15 and my mother gave me the Benefit High Beam Highlighter. I went straight to the bathroom to play (still my favourite pastime after all these years!) but I got myself in a right pickle as I was wearing an extraordinary amount of Rimmel Stay Matte powder. I could very clearly see stripe marks where I hadn't blended and it had congealed in the copious amounts of powder and downy hair on my face. It wasn't a great look BUT I studied it intensely, quickly learnt what not to do and had perfected my glow in no time!

Powder highlighters

Powder highlighters are an excellent option for those who consider themselves slightly oily and don't want to add any unnecessary moisture to the skin. They do, however, vary greatly in quality. There are some exquisite powders that are so finely milled that they look and feel more like cream, whereas some are flaky with heavy particles that will feel dry and sit unflatteringly and almost patchily on the skin. I recommend you do a swatch before you buy. If that's not possible, do an online search as makeup enthusiasts are quick to share their opinions online, which can be incredibly helpful and, of course, don't forget to check the reviews on the product's website too.

When applying powder highlight, I prefer to use a small-headed fluffy brush, mainly so I don't apply too much. A dense brush will cause too intense a finish, so a lightly bound brush head is best. When dipping into your powder highlight, be careful not to pick up too much product. It's far easier to pick up a tiny bit and build the luminosity than it is to try to take down too much shimmer.

LIQUID HIGHLIGHTERS I LIKE:

– Iconic London Illuminator

– Charlotte Tilbury Hollywood Flawless Filter

– Beauty Pie Triple Beauty Luminizing Wand

– Vieve Skin Nova

– Illamasqua Beyond Liquid Highlighter

– Sculpted By Aimee Liquid Lights

POWDER HIGHLIGHTERS I LIKE:

– Charlotte Tilbury Hollywood Glow Glide Face Architect Highlighter

– Ciaté Glow-To Highlighter

– Hourglass Ambient Strobe Lighting Powder

– Illamasqua Beyond Powder Highlighter

– Kiko Ultimate Glow Highlighter

– Revolution Super Highlight

APPLICATION TIP

Just like with blush and bronzer, I recommend tapping the powder into the head of the brush by tapping the brush head into the palm of your hand. This will ensure you don't have too many metallic pigments on your brush that may be tricky to blend out.

Load the brush head with the highlighter and gradually build. If you create too great an area of highlight, you lose the lifting benefit of using the highlighter and simply create great swathes of shimmer, rather than using the light reflection to illuminate certain areas and bring them to the forefront. I do recommend you blend your highlighter with a clean brush once you have applied it.

As already stated, I love the all-over glow effect achieved by applying a highlighter over the face underneath foundation. However, you can use highlighter to spot light key areas, such as the top of the cheek, the bridge of the nose, along the brow bone, the cupid's bow and the temples.

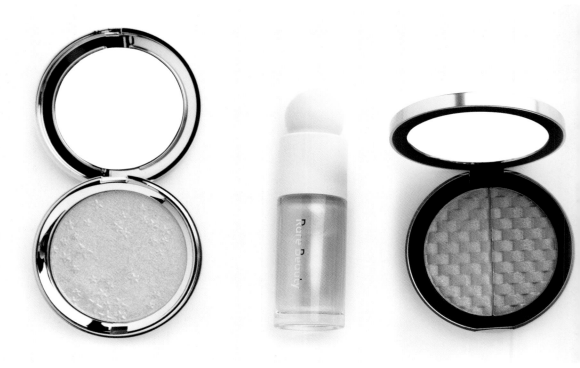

Cream highlighters

Cream highlighter is probably my favourite to work with. I love being able to tap it into the skin with my fingers and melt the cream into whatever base products I've applied underneath. A cream in a pan or stick allows me to have more control, and there is potentially less room for error.

> *I find having different formulas in my kit is essential so that I have the right highlighter for any client, but I also use different textures for various things.*

For example, I may use a liquid highlighter under foundation for a soft focus glow, cream highlighter on the very top of the cheekbones as a finishing touch and the tiniest bit of powder highlighter under the browbone (this is because it will wear better than a cream or liquid and I'm able to get finer, more precise application in this area with a powder and a very fine brush).

CREAM HIGHLIGHTERS I LIKE:

– Westman Atelier Super Loaded Tinted Highlight

– Trinny London The Right Light Highlighter

– RMS Beauty Magic Luminiser

– Sculpted By Aimee Cream Luxe Glow

– Illamasqua Gleam Highlighter

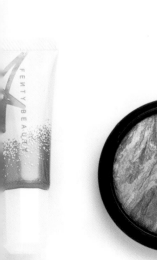

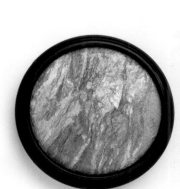

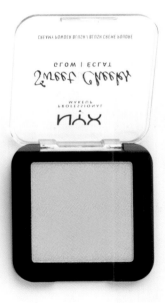

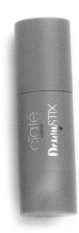

GLITTER

Of course I had to have a glitter section! I absolutely love it.

> *For daytime, weddings, black-tie events – any occasion – glitter can simply bring a little bit of joy!*

I understand glitter isn't for everyone and if you're not a fan, that's totally ok, we can still be friends, but sparkle played a huge part in igniting my love of makeup. There was a shop in the nearest town to where I grew up and they had a fairly small makeup display by a brand called Spectacular. They made multicoloured wash-in, wash-out hair dye (my sister had purple-and-blue hair for quite some time), nail varnish, pots of glitter pigment, glitter lipsticks (yaaaaaassssss) and glitter hair spray. My friends and I would paw these cosmetics for hours and buy bits here and there when budgets allowed and, my goodness, the joy I felt when wearing my glitter lipstick or my glitter hairspray. It was such an uplifting feeling that glitter has remained a firm favourite in both my personal and professional kit.

I know some worry about the age-appropriateness of glitter, but I honestly think you're never too old for a little sparkle – you may just want to alter the texture slightly for a more flattering finish.

Twenty years ago the offerings were fairly minimal, with chunky glitter that often fell from the eyes and went everywhere because it was too heavy to adhere to the skin, or bizarre roll-on glitter gels that really only belonged at festivals. It's a different story now, with numerous offerings of beautifully finely milled, biodegradable glitter particles in shadows that not only adhere better because they're so small and light, but also lay over the skin with no 'background' colour, so they don't emphasise the appearance of fine lines on the lid like some metallic shadows might.

I mention this as some might think that a metallic shadow could be a 'safer' alternative to glitter, but I'd argue that delicate glitter is much more flattering than metallic shadow. Metallic shadow can get caught in fine lines and reflect light in such a way that it highlights the folds in the skin.

GLITTER I LIKE:

– Urban Decay Heavy Metal Glitter Liner

– Nabla Glorious Lights

– MAC Reflects Glitter

– NYX Professional Makeup Metallic Eye Glitter

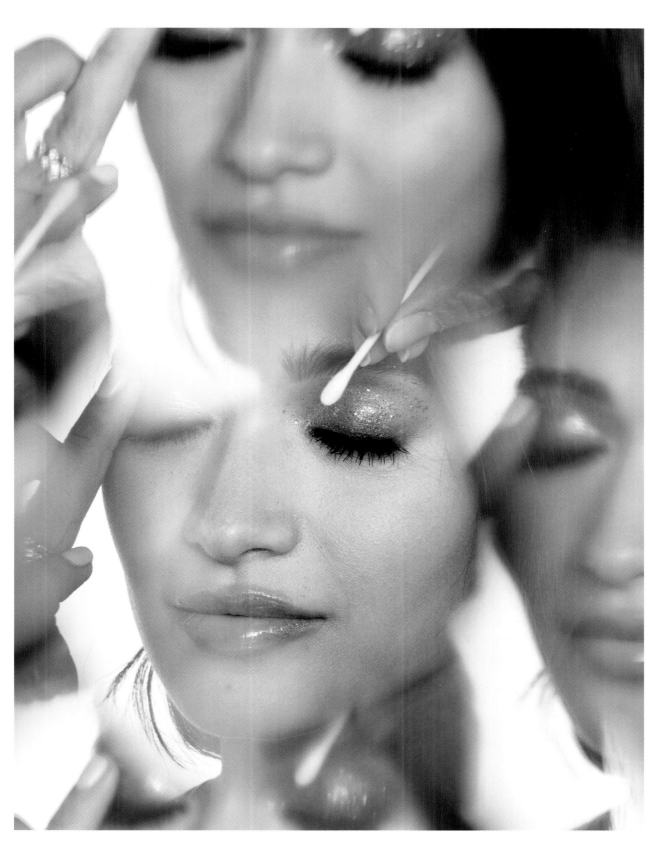

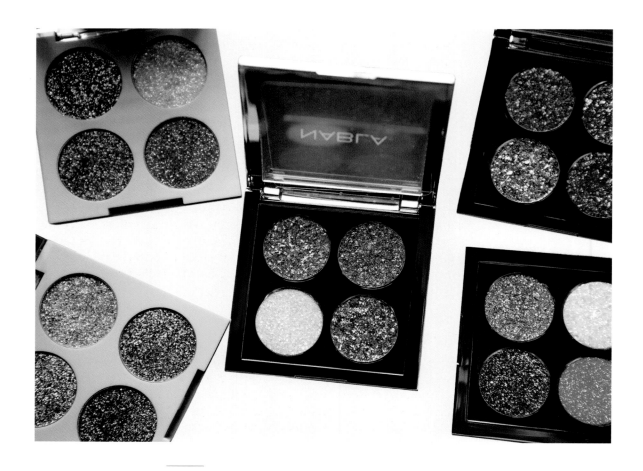

APPLICATION

> *A simple sparkle pigment pressed into the centre of the lid with your ring finger as a finishing touch can beautifully elevate any makeup look on anyone of any age.*

Using your finger will prevent fall out (when makeup drops from the eyes onto the cheek) as glitter pigment in the bristles of a brush can fall when the brush moves or can be flicked out of the brush when the bristles brush past your lashes.

It's much more effective to 'press and sweep' with your fingers. The reason I write 'press and sweep' is that you do need to move your fingertip once it's in contact with the skin to lay down the glitter, but only a little. I see people 'dabbing' their sparkle pigment and, unfortunately, you'll only get a little of the pigment from your finger onto the lid as the particles love to adhere to skin. For effective, long-lasting lay down, you need to press your finger onto the skin and 'dab and sweep' in small motions of only just a few millimetres at a time.

It can also be helpful if you press a little glitter through the crease of the eye to help diffuse the edge of a smokey eye. The optical illusion of the twinkle of a few sparkle pigments softens and blurs the finish of the shadow.

I sometimes apply a little glitter to the top of the cheeks too, usually in place of highlighter, and I find the tiniest touch can be really alluring and often cause people to ask 'Ooooh, what's that on your cheek?' The key, as I previously stated, is the size of the glitter itself. If you want it to be subtle, go small; if you want all-out disco, then go for lots of different-sized glitters for a multi-dimensional dazzle.

FORMATS

Whilst my preference is for pressed glitter in the pan, you can get loose glitter pigments in pots and glitter in gels and eyeliners. If you opt for loose pigment, do your eyes first to prevent the glitter falling into your makeup. Alternatively, you can hold a tissue under your eyes as you apply the glitter to catch the fall out. Gosh, I just had a major flashback to uni when I worked in nightclubs and glitter was my go-to. This was exactly how I applied my glitter shadow. I bought it on Oxford Street – my friend Holly and I made cheap trips on the bus to London especially to go glitter shopping!

GLITTER FALL OUT

If you do get glitter fall out that you'd like to get rid of, then a spoolie wand can be a great tool for flicking away unwanted particles from the skin, as are firm mascara fan brushes. For any stubborn ones, a piece of white-tac or scotch tape works wonders – it's just usually my last resort as there is risk of moving the makeup underneath.

Whilst glitter may not be to everyone's taste, I hope that for anyone reading this who assumed that glitter was just for teenagers may have been persuaded to think otherwise and give it a go.

BRUSHES

BRUSHES

The right tools can make your job so much easier. This is as true when it comes to makeup as it is for a chef and his kitchen knives, or a golfer and his clubs.

> *Often when clients of mine have been struggling with a technique, a lot of the issues can be attributed to the tool they're trying to achieve the look with.*

Let's take blush, for example. If you're trying to achieve a subtle flush to the cheek but you only have a large powder brush, then you're going to struggle to get precise placement. You will end up with too much blush on too great a surface of the cheek.

The same goes for eyeshadow. If you're trying to achieve something delicate but your brushes are big and cumbersome, it's not going to happen.

There are literally hundreds of thousands of brushes on the market and I'm constantly trying out new ones, but like most makeup artists, I have a few that I come back to time and time again!

Skincare

Some people like to use brushes for skincare. I'm a firm believer in using fingers to apply skincare as I love manipulating the products in my fingers and using the warmth of my hands to help work them into the skin, but that's not everyone's preference and these days it's not always allowed on clients.

During the pandemic, when I was allowed to work, which was minimal (though television jobs could go ahead), I had to retrain myself to apply products with tools as I had to wear gloves at all times. And you definitely can't apply products with gloves on! So, whilst my preference will always be hands, synthetic flat foundation brushes are excellent for applying serums, moisturisers and SPF.

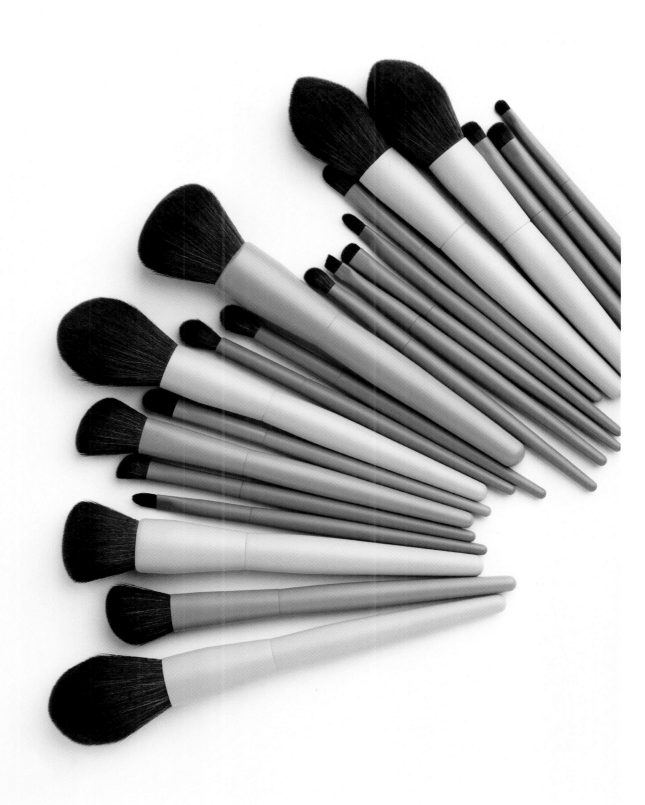

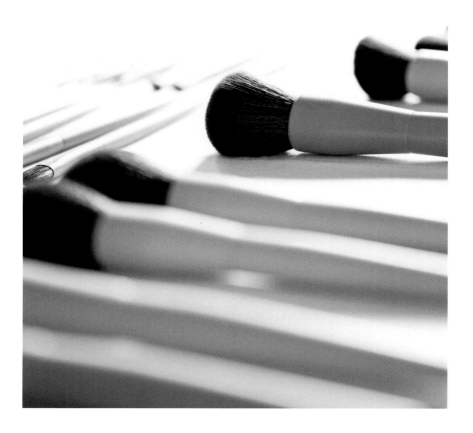

WHY YOU SHOULD USE SYNTHETIC BRUSHES

1 I believe all brushes should be synthetic. Even though I know lots of natural hair brushes don't harm the animals they come from, it makes no sense to not use synthetic in this day and age.

2 These days, synthetic fibres can be so fine that there really is little difference between them and natural brushes (not like the cumbersome, thick plastic bristles of previous brushes).

3 Synthetic fibres don't absorb moisture like natural hair does. If you try to apply any cream product with a natural hair brush, you'll have some level of success, but actually you'll probably find that the brush is absorbing a lot of your product. A synthetic fibre will carry the product, then allow you to lay it onto the skin more effectively, preventing product waste.

I know some like to use fluffy brushes, but I find I have more control when using a traditional flat-headed foundation brush. You can apply light pressure to work the product into the skin, whereas fluffy brushes just lay the product on the surface.

MUAs also use sponges to apply skincare, which is fine, but I prefer to use skincare on a sponge as more of a fixing technique rather than as a means of application. I think sponges became popular in recent years thanks to their use on social media, with artists on YouTube and Instagram using them and teaching the younger generation their practices.

Call me old school, but hands work best for me.

Quick side note:
I always have a towel laid out on the surface where I am doing my makeup for three reasons: so the products don't roll around, it's quieter when setting products down and so I can wipe my fingers and brushes between use. If you find yourself going through endless tissues, a hand towel or flannel can be useful – just be sure to wash them frequently.

FLAT FOUNDATION BRUSHES I LIKE:

— Armani Beauty Foundation Brush

— Clé de Peau Beauté Foundation Brush

— Lisa Eldridge No1 The Foundation Brush

— Morphe M707 Foundation Brush

— MAC 190 Foundation Brush

— Hannah Martin x Ciaté Base Brush #1

— MyKitCo My Smoothing Foundation

— Joy Adenuga Multi-use Face Brush 005

How to use a sponge to correct texture

1 First soak the sponge in water until it's almost doubled in size, then wring out the water until there are no drips. The act of soaking the sponge will stop it absorbing too much of your product.

2 Pick up a little moisturiser with a cotton bud and work into the sponge.

3 Bounce the sponge lightly over the face to take off any excess makeup and ease the appearance of texture. By texture, I mean any makeup that's looking a little congealed. This can happen on areas of dryness or blemishes, so by adding the tiniest bit of skincare to the makeup, it magically brings it back to life.

You can use a hydrating mist, but it's harder to treat small surface areas and it doesn't help lift off excess makeup.

Foundation brushes

There are many tools for applying foundation but the five most common are:

- **Fingertips**
- **Flat foundation brushes**
- **Fluffy foundation brushes**
- **Firm flat-headed foundation brushes**
- **Sponges**

Often you can create a sheerer finish if you simply use your fingertips to apply your base. A dab of foundation on the forehead, each cheek, nose and chin, and then blended with the fingers works wonders and is exactly how my mother applied her base all those years I sat watching at her feet.

However, I have regularly witnessed on public transport for the 16-plus years I've been living in London, people applying foundation as if it were moisturiser – huge, great amounts rubbed in, fairly vigorously and repeatedly, until blended. In this case, it is easy to overdo the base and use more than you need . . .

With **flat foundation brushes**, I recommend popping the foundation into the palm of your hand and using it a bit like a palette.

Quick side note:
For any MUAs reading, a mixing plate or palette is key to reduce the risk of cross-contamination.

Dip the tip of the brush into the product and start blending from the centre of the face out. I generally start around the nose as many people carry a little redness here. Once this redness is corrected with a little base, it can be all you need to do when it comes to base makeup application.

If it's a full makeup look you're going for, then continue to apply the base products over the entire face using both sides of the brush and blending with lots of repetitive strokes. Don't go back and forth with the brush, use short strokes to go over the same area a few times.

*

Stipple:
This is the act of applying products in tiny dots and brush movements that blend for a flawless finish.

Non-comedogenic:
This is a skincare product that aims not to block your pores.

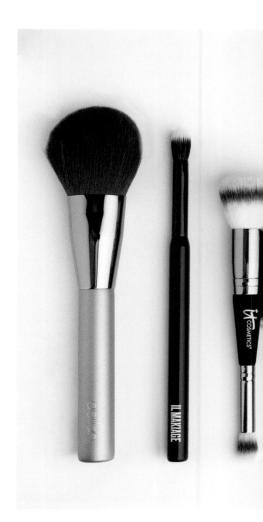

STRIPY OR STREAKY FOUNDATION

If you find your foundation is looking a little stripy or streaky, this is usually an indication that your foundation brush needs cleaning and has gone a bit firm due to product build-up. In an ideal world, you'd wash a flat foundation brush after each use (this is of course a must if it's your work brush) but once a week is ok – any longer than that and you'll find your bristles go firm and you won't get the finish you're looking for.

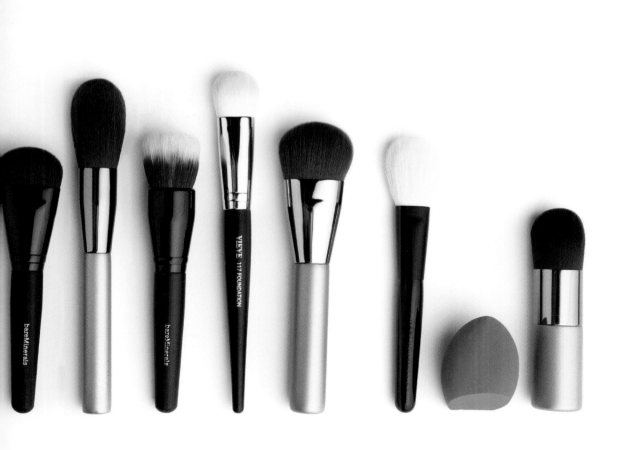

With **fluffy foundation brushes**, you get a much lighter base application as the bristles are a lot less densely bound. They're a great option if you're using a tinted moisturiser or another light base. I often use a small fluffy brush to apply foundation when I'm working on shoots as, more often than not, beauty models have glorious skin and don't need much makeup. So, if you're not looking for full coverage, give a fluffy-headed brush a whirl.

Pump the base product into the palm of your hand (or onto a palette if working on someone else), dip the tip of the brush in and work the product into the brush by swirling it around on the back of your hand. This will ensure the base product is evenly distributed in the brush hairs and will make application that bit more even.

Applying foundation directly to the brush

It's a craze on social media to apply foundation directly to the brush head or sponge. Whilst it's not wrong per se and everyone has their preferred way of applying their base, it's not something I teach. It can be all kinds of messy and, more importantly, you may find you apply much more product than you need.

By taking a little bit of base at a time from your hand or palette to your brush, you can build up the coverage bit by bit and have a little more control.

With a smaller, fluffy brush, I tend to apply foundation in a much more delicate way – small motions back and forth, applying very little pressure, often in sweeping and circular motions whilst keeping the brush head in contact with the skin.

The focus here is on light coverage that's so well-blended it's almost undetectable. I'll often use the same brush for gel bronzer and blush for these reasons too. For creams, I prefer slightly firmer brushes as they help blend and move the product more efficiently.

ROUNDED FOUNDATION BRUSHES I LIKE:

- Beauty Pie Foundation Buffing Brush

- bareMinerals Smoothing Face Brush

- IT Cosmetics Heavenly Luxe Complexion Brush

- Bobbi Brown Full Coverage Face Brush

- Vieve 117 Foundation Brush

- Real Techniques Expert Face Brush

- Charlotte Tilbury Complexion Brush

- NYX Professional Makeup Pro Multi-Purpose Buffing Brush

- Anastasia Beverly Hills A30 Brush

- Huda Face Buff & Blend Brush

- Shiseido Daiya Fude Brush

- Hourglass Vanish Seamless Finish Foundation Brush

- Refy Duo Brush

- Hannah Martin x Ciaté Base Brush #2

- MyKitCo My Flawless Foundation Brush

Firm flat-headed foundation brushes – the kind that are usually round in shape and cut flat, but can be angled – I use for more full-coverage makeup looks and a lot for cream contour. A densely bound foundation brush is usually made up of thousands of synthetic brush hairs that help you to evenly distribute and blend foundation for a full-cover finish, so I love to use these with heavier, more pigmented foundations that are usually a little thicker in texture and so need more work to blend.

Again, I'd recommend dipping the tip of the brush into your full-coverage foundation and to start blending from the cheek to get a sense of how the foundation looks and feels. Alternatively, dot the full-coverage foundation over the cheeks, forehead, nose and chin and then blend with the flat-headed foundation brush.

These brushes don't work so well with lighter bases as the hairs are so dense that they either lift off or absorb more sheer, emollient bases, which is frustrating and wasteful. Stick to your looser brushes for those. I also really like the ability to stipple with a firm flat-headed foundation brush. I add in a few circular motions when applying and then tap really lightly, pushing the very tips of the bristles into the base to blend, but also to ensure there are no obvious brush strokes and to help disguise the appearance of pores.

PORES HACK

I find that stippling a brush over the cheeks, chin and forehead, or anywhere where there may be slightly larger pores, helps to work makeup into the skin and therefore smooth over the pores. In fact, when I can, I'll stipple with the brush and then press gently with my fingertips to melt the makeup into the skin further. If you just sweep a foundation over open pores, it can sit rather obviously on the surface of the skin and you can exacerbate their appearance.

Thankfully, with advances in makeup technology, most foundations are non-comedogenic and won't cause the pores to become blocked. But you should always remove makeup thoroughly. You may have heard of double cleansing – essentially the act of cleansing twice. This can be with the same product or with different ones and this is something I highly recommend for those that wear full-coverage makeup, as you can miss so much when just cleansing once.

SPONGES I LIKE:

– Beauty Blender

– Real Techniques Miracle Complexion Sponge

– Beauty Bay Microfibre Sponge

– Tarte Quickie Blending Sponge

– Kylie Cosmetics Makeup Sponge

– LH Cosmetics The Sponge

– Fenty Beauty Precision Makeup Sponge

– Iconic London Seamless Blender

– Boots Cosmetic Sponge Wedges (for detail)

VELOUR PUFFS I LIKE:

– Laura Mercier Velour Puff

– LH Cosmetics The Powder Puff

– Beautyblender Powder Puff

– Makeup Forever Ultra HD Setting Powder Puff

– MyKitCo My Deluxe Puffs

– Kryolan Premium Powder Puff

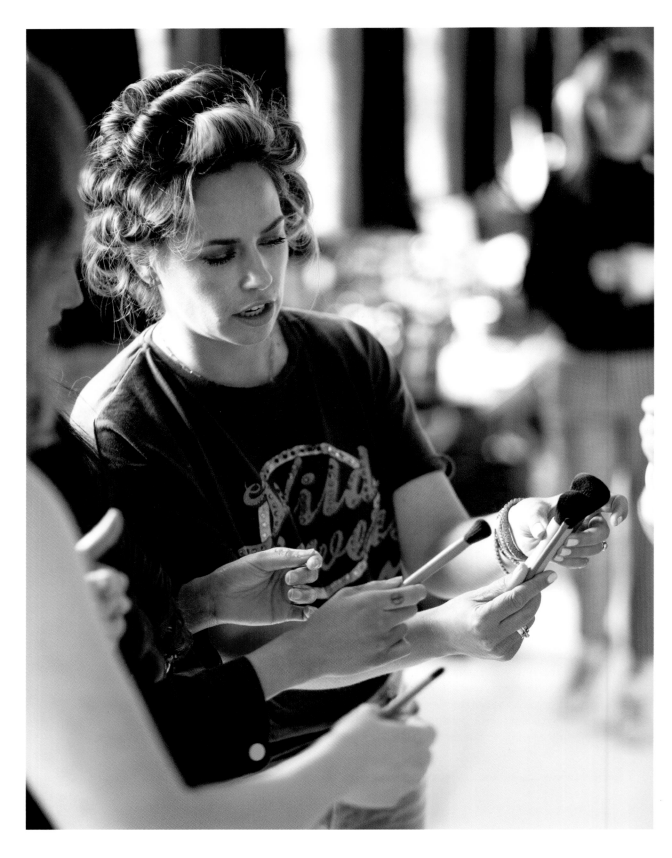

CONTOUR

I'll use a firm flat-headed foundation brush for cream contour and firmer cream blushers because they help lay down the product and give you great control over placement. For contour, for example, you want to place it in very specific areas initially, which you then blend out. For powder contour, which I do after all the cream-based products have been applied and usually at the end of a makeup session to enhance the cream contour, I use a much lighter, **loosely bound powder brush** as a softer applicator. Too firm a brush will create a striped effect.

> *Firm brushes for cream contour, loose, fluffy brushes for finishing touches in powder contour.*

Sponges are best soaked in lukewarm water before use so that they are more supple and won't absorb too much of your product. As I've said, the trend currently is to pump foundation onto the tip of the sponge, but guess what I'm going to say? No prizes here:

> *I prefer to dot my foundation first or dip into the foundation on my palm or palette and then bounce the sponge over the face.*

Yes, bounce! That is the best technique when it comes to sponge application. I see people sweeping and swiping with sponges but the real beauty of the sponge is the ability to bounce it over your makeup with lots and lots of light-handed dabs. This will blend all textures of base makeup over the face, from skincare to tinted moisturiser to your fullest-coverage base.

> *The bounce blends makeup evenly and gently.*

It makes sense to fully blend out each area as you apply, rather than bouncing from, say, your cheek to your forehead to your chin and then back. If you do this, you can end up with a patchy-looking base and areas of fuller coverage than others, so I suggest starting on your cheek and fully blending out that area. I tend to bounce in a small circle initially, then gradually widen the circle to distribute the product. I then follow over to the nose, then to the other cheek before doing the chin and forehead. True of all makeup application, this more methodical approach ensures the most even finish.

CONTOUR BRUSHES I LIKE:

- Charlotte Tilbury Powder and Sculpt Brush

- Beauty Pie Pro Angled Contour Cheek Brush

- Look Good Feel Better Angled Contour Brush

- Illamasqua Contouring Brush

- Hannah Martin x Ciaté Small Powder

- Hannah Martin x Ciaté Tiny Eye/Face Contour 1

- Hannah Martin x Ciaté Tiny Eye/Face Contour 2

- Morphe E62 Angled Nose Contouring

- Zoeva 130 Luxe Contour Definer

- Huda Beauty Dual-Ended Contour and Bronze Complexion Brush

- Daniel Sandler Sculpt/Contour Brush

- Smith Cosmetics Black 124 Contour Brush

Most sponges are teardrop shaped, allowing you to manipulate them to make the most of all its angles. I use the flatter bottom of the sponge to do most of the foundation work, but then the finer-pointed tip for under the eyes and around the nose.

MINI SPONGES FOR UNDER THE EYE

Sponges come in all shapes and sizes and I really like the teeny little sponges. I use these to help blend out concealer under the eye, especially on more mature skin that can feel quite loose and where finger taps don't work as well. You can push the very slim tip of a small sponge into the concealer and not disturb the skin too much.

Thank you, Tanya Cropsey, for that tip!

Sponges can be used for techniques like baking and some like to spray their sponges with setting spray and bounce over the base instead of spritzing. It works but is something to do cautiously as, of course, the risk here is inadvertently lifting the makeup beneath if you apply too much pressure with the sponge. This method works best with lighter coverage looks.

Whilst many use their sponge to apply just about everything, I still prefer to use them in the main as a blending tool. They're brilliant for buffing makeup edges and making sure the blend of your blush into your bronzer, for example, is smooth.

If you're someone who at the end of their makeup application worries that it looks heavy or patchy, then you could benefit from a makeup sponge as the last step in your routine to seamlessly blend your products together.

Concealer brushes

There are lots of options for brushes to use for concealer, but I've always loved quite a **long, flat brush** to apply at least the first few strokes of concealer. A long, flat brush allows you to get right into the inner corner of the eye and under the lower lashes to get a bit of product onto the skin.

Once I've done that, I recommend using a **light fluffy brush**, like a MAC 217, which is possibly more commonly used as a crease shadow brush, to distribute the product. Alternatively, I use the pad of my finger to press the concealer into the skin.

With my clients, I often use a **corrector** first to make sure the under eye is as bright and clean as possible. Use a **flat concealer brush** to apply that, then blend with your finger.

I then use a **fluffier brush** for the **skin tone-correct concealer** I apply on top. I will say that a fluffy brush works wonders on beautiful models with barely any under-eye shadows and no saggy skin, but it can be tricky with more mature eyes that have some loose skin. I suggest those that feel they need concealer to have both brushes to work with.

You can of course use **sponges** to apply concealer, too, in which case it's a similar motion to your foundation blending – a mixture of gentle tapping and wiping to get the concealer exactly where you want it.

FLAT CONCEALER BRUSHES I LIKE:

– Bobbi Brown Concealer Blending Brush

– Morphe M224 Oval Camouflage Brush

– bareMinerals Maximum Coverage Concealer Brush

– Clé de Peau Beauté Concealer Brush

– Laura Mercier Secret Camouflage Brush

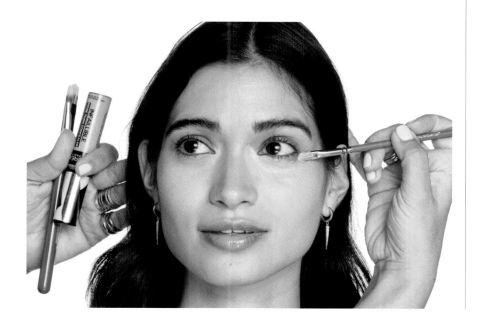

Concealing blemishes

Ideally, you'd let a blemish heal entirely before applying makeup in that area – that's the best thing to aid their healing, especially if you've picked at it. However, I suggest how best to conceal here as I know that sometimes you might have an occasion or event that you want to attend.

If you're looking to conceal blemishes, then I recommend using a **flat brush** first, sanitised of course, and draw an 'x' over the blemish in question. Then use a **smaller domed concealer brush** to stipple the concealer into place.

Make sure the concealer you're using to conceal any blemishes is the same shade as your foundation. If you use under-eye concealer (which is usually a little lighter) you could be highlighting the thing you're trying to hide.

Once the concealer is blended, set it in place with some powder. I recommend stippling translucent loose powder on a small brush over the concealer to lock it in place. This method is so helpful when wanting to really work concealer into the skin but especially if you're working with a scab or broken skin that isn't flat, as you need to be able to get the product into all the creases.

Please don't think I'm saying you must cover blemishes – you absolutely don't – but this is how I recommend you do it if you want to.

If you get a cold sore, again, they are best left alone but if you're desperate to conceal one, then decant some of your concealer onto the back of your hand, dip the tip of a cotton bud into it and press that over the cold sore. Just be sure to never dip the cotton bud into the actual product as you don't want to contaminate it, then also throw the used tip away immediately.

FLUFFY CONCEALER BRUSHES I LIKE:

– e.l.f. Flawless Concealer Brush

– MyKitCo 0.3 My Fluffy Concealer Brush

– Illamasqua Round Concealer Brush

– Real Techniques 402

– Nars Radiant Creamy Concealer Brush

– Urban Decay Pro Domed Concealer Brush

DOMED CONCEALER BRUSHES I LIKE:

– Bobbi Brown Touch Up Brush

– Real Techniques 210 Expert Concealer

– Zoeva 145 Concealer Blender

– Zoeva 146 Concealer Perfector

– Hourglass Vanish Seamless Finish Concealer Brush

– Morphe M173 Chubby Buffer

Powder brushes

I use powder with either a **big brush**, a **little brush**, a **puff** or a **sponge**.

If you like to use powder to set your makeup, then a great big powder brush will make your task quick and easy.

POWDER HACK

The key is to make sure you tap the powder, not your brush, so you load the brush head with product rather than leaving the pigment sitting on the tip of your brush. This prevents you ending up with a great big blob of powder wherever your brush first makes contact with the skin. Whilst that's not the end of the world, it can look a bit patchy, with some areas more matte and powdery than others.

POWDER BRUSHES I LIKE:

– bareMinerals Supreme Finisher Brush

– Morphe E3 Precision Pointed Powder Brush and E2 Powder Brush

– Real Techniques Powder Brush

– Zoeva 106 Powder Brush

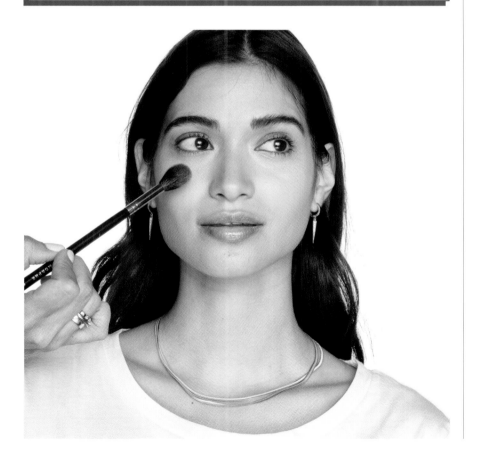

You can lightly sweep the powder brush over the face for a light set or stipple the powder in for a more matte, full-cover set.

I also have lots of medium and dinky sizes of **loosely bound powder brushes** for the times I don't want too much powder applied, whether that's because I'm looking for a more dewy finish or because I'm just wanting to set makeup in certain areas. For under the eyes, around the nose and between the brows, you need a much smaller-headed brush or you're going to magnify a greater surface area than desired.

Velour pads and **sponges** are also effective for use with setting powder, specifically if you're looking to eliminate as much shine as possible.

I prefer to not use a sponge for my setting powder (though I may use it to bake under my contour as previously mentioned) but you can use your sponge to apply powder if you like.

Much like with foundation, tip a bit of your loose powder into the palm of your hand, dip the sponge into the powder and then bounce the powder over the area you want to set or mattify. Just be careful that your sponge isn't wet from any skincare or base product you may have used it for previously. I know lots of MUAs use different-coloured sponges for different things to avoid any confusion: white for skincare, pink for foundation and black for powder, for example.

TV makeup

If I'm working with someone for a television appearance and not for a glossy red-carpet moment, then I'll get out my trusty **velour puff** and really press the powder into the makeup. I usually roll the puff around my index and middle finger, then roll the pad loaded with powder over the skin.

It's best to be really methodical in your application here so you create the same depth of matte finish all over. If you pat sporadically from the chin to the nose to the forehead to the cheek again, you run the risk of a patchy finish, so I'll do the forehead first, then focus on and around the nose, then the front of the cheeks, ending with the chin.

Blush brushes

For blush, I think it's key to have a brush designed specifically for blush application. There are lots of brushes I use for multiple products, but I don't think blush is one of them, as placement is so important.

Really, the best blush tools are your fingers for liquids and creams, very small fluffy brushes for liquids, firm flat brushes for creams and angled, loosely bound brushes for powder. You can use a sponge, too, of course, for cream-based blush.

I have a couple of treasured blush brushes that I absolutely love, that are cut in a way that gives me brilliant control over where I place the blush.

While lots of blush brush heads are long and domed at the tip, I much prefer a brush cut on an angle to really hug the apple of the cheek. If a blush brush head is too big, you won't get the same precise finish and can risk applying too much colour to too large an area.

For creams, I do like to use fingers, but for liquid blush, I think a very small, synthetic brush is best as you need something very loosely bound or the brush will lift the product straight off again.

To get an even blend with a powder blush, it's best to use a loosely bound fluffy brush. If the brush is too dense, you may find your blush application is too dense and the pigment too strong.

> *When it comes to blush, it's much easier to add colour by layering than it is to try to buff away too strong a blush.*

BLUSH BRUSHES I LIKE:

– Hannah Martin x Ciaté Blush Brush

– Bobbi Brown Blush Brush

– Bobbi Brown Angled Face Brush

– Joy Adenuga Multi-use 012

– Shiseido Maru Fude Multi Face Brush

– Smith Cosmetics 118 Blush/Powder Brush

– Morphe R46 Cream and Powder Blush Brush

– Spectrum MA05 Angled Cheek Brush

– Nars Blush Brush

– Hourglass Blush Brush

– Laura Mercier Cheek Color Brush

– Charlotte Tilbury Bronzer and Blusher Brush

Bronzer brushes

When it comes to bronzer, there are a few brushes I reach for time and time again: a **large, flat-headed, loosely bound bronzer brush**, a **large powder brush** and a synthetic **flat-headed foundation brush** for bronzing creams and gels.

· **For bronzing gels**, a **really light, fluffy synthetic brush** is all you need, as you want it to lay the product on the skin gently and almost allow it to stain.

· With **creams**, a **firmer brush** is helpful to move the product around the skin effectively.

· For **powder**, I use a **large fluffy brush** to create the most naturally bronzed effect, as you want to diffuse the pigment across a fairly large area. A smaller brush will take you longer to do this and you run the risk of creating bronzer stripes.

· A more even finish and avoiding bronzer stripes is also why I prefer **flat-headed bronzer brushes** to dome-cut to pointed powder brushes.

I remember the first time I was backstage working with Bobbi Brown at the *Lorraine* show on TV here in the UK. I was applying a model's bronzer and Bobbi kept saying, 'More Hannah, more,' because the model's body was so much warmer than her face and neck. And, of course, a larger brush was the most efficient way of doing this. I think before then I had always exercised a little too much caution but now, whilst I never want to overdo it, I confidently apply bronzer until I see the skin's tone is all in colour harmony and shaded correctly,

It's key to note here that while this is what I generally recommend, there will always be exceptions to the rule and people will have preferences for different tools, just as they do with products. So, it may be that you prefer to apply bronzer with a smaller brush. That's fine and can be necessary in some cases, for example, those with very fine, dainty features.

Highlighter brushes

For highlighter, I recommend a fluffy, loosely bound, small powder brush. I may use one as small as the Bobbi Brown Eye Blender Brush, to ensure I don't apply too much product and have control over its placement. If applying highlighter with too big a brush you may spread it much further than intended and you won't achieve the 'spot-lit' look you're aiming for.

BRONZER BRUSHES I LIKE:

– Bobbi Brown Bronzer Brush

– Hannah Martin x Ciaté Bronzer Brush

– Clé de Peau Beauté Bronzer Brush

– Zoeva 119 Bronzer Brush

– Spectrum A01 Domed Powder Brush

– Fenty Beauty Face Shaping Brush 125

– Iconic London Ultimate Bronzing Brush

– Morphe M611 Bronze Show Fluffy Bronzer Brush

HIGHLIGHTER BRUSHES I LIKE:

– Real Techniques 402

– Bobbi Brown Eye Blender Brush

– bareMinerals Diffused Highlighter Brush

– Hourglass Detail Setting Brush

– Morphe M501 Pointed Blender Highlighter

– Smashbox Precise Highlighting Brush

– Zoeva 134 Luxe Powder Fusion Brush

Eyeshadow brushes

There are so many brushes available when it comes to eyeshadow, so here are the top ones that I think are the most useful to have.

- **Classic eyeshadow brush**
- **Fluffier brush for crease colour and blending**
- **Small-headed, firmer, synthetic, flat shadow brush for creams**
- **Flat-domed brush for detail and smudging**
- **Thin, flat brush for both powder and gel eyeliner**

There are numerous options in each category, my favourites of which I list below, but I think these are the most essential when it comes to creating most eye looks and should make up the most basic kit.

EYESHADOW BRUSHES I LIKE:

Base colour:

- Bobbi Brown Eye Sweep Brush
- Kevyn Aucoin The Base Shadow Brush
- bareMinerals Shade & Diffuse Eye Brush
- Hourglass No 3 All Over Shadow Brush
- Shiseido Naname Fude Multi Eye Brush
- Hannah Martin x Ciaté Flat Eye base
- Hannah Martin x Ciaté Fluffy Eye Base
- MAC 287 Duo Fibre Eyeshadow Brush
- Louise Young LY39 V Domed Shadow Brush

Lid colour:

- Hannah Martin x Ciaté Eye Detail Brush
- Bobbi Brown Eyeshadow Brush
- Morphe X Ariel A29
- Morphe M166 Oval Shadow
- Louise Young LY10 V Flat Shadow Brush
- Louise Young LY18 V Classic Shadow Brush
- Fenty Beauty Plush Eyeshadow Brush 240
- Zoeva 222 Luxe All Over Shader Brush
- Zoeva 239 Luxe Soft Shader Brush
- MAC 252S Large Shader Brush

Fluffy crease colour/ Blending:

- Hannah Martin x Ciaté Crease/ Blending 1
- Hannah Martin x Ciaté Crease/ Blending 2
- MAC 217
- Vieve 219/219 Small Eyeshadow Blender
- Charlotte Tilbury Eye Blender Brush
- Zoeva 228 Luxe Crease Brush
- Zoeva 224 Luxe Defined Crease Brush
- Spectrum Mini Tapered Blender B10
- Spectrum Tall Crease Blender MB07
- Morphe M433 Firm Blending Fluff Eyeshadow

- Morphe M573 Pointed Deluxe Blender
- Morphe M330 Blending Crease Eyeshadow
- Morphe M513 Round Blender
- Louise Young LY38 V Tapered Shadow Brush

Detail:

- Bobbi Brown Smokey Eyeliner Brush
- Hannah Martin x Ciaté Smudger
- Hannah Martin x Ciaté Small Smudge
- Louise Young LY38B V Slim Tapered Shadow Brush
- Louise Young LY08 V Small Detail Brush
- Louise Young LY13 V Mini Socket Brush
- Louise Young LY16 V Mini Smudge Brush
- Morphe M431 Precision Pencil Crease
- Morphe M514 Detail Round Blender Eyeshadow
- Morphe M149 Small Round Contour
- Morphe M321 Bullet Crease Eyeshadow Brush

Brow brushes

Brow brushes are most commonly slim and cut on an angle. The essential versions are:

• **Spoolie wand**
• **Slim angled brush**
• **Firmer angled brush**

If a brow brush is too soft, it can 'splay' and disperse the powder across too great an area, which is not what you want when trying to create natural-looking, brow-like strokes with your powder. A firm brush is best as it only places the powder exactly where you put it.

The **spoolie** is needed to comb your brows before makeup application but they're also excellent for brushing out your brows once they're done and softening any pencil strokes for a more natural finish.

Slim brow brushes cut on an angle are ideal for gels and pomades as you can coat them in product and then perfect the tip by dabbing each side on the back of your hand or over the lip of the pomade pot to ensure the bristles are all grouped together and neat and slim. This will help you to draw in very fine hairs.

I always use a **firmer angled brush**, like the Bobbi Brown Dual-Ended Brow Brush. I hope they never change this as it's the only one I have of its kind and it works amazingly with powder brows. It's really firm and quite coarse, which works so well.

NEATENING UP AN UNEVEN BROW

A **slim concealer brush** can be helpful to conceal around the brows to neaten up an uneven brow line. Apply a bit of concealer right beneath the brow line to make your brows look more uniform.

Usually people do this as a finishing touch, but I sometimes create an earlier step where I use a little concealer under the brows, say if someone has scarring in the area or uneven skin that can affect how the brow products translate. Sometimes brow powders don't adhere to softer scar tissue, and a bit of concealer gives the product something to stick to. So, place a little concealer along the brow bone, blend it out and then perfect with the brow product. A smaller brush is helpful as the area you're looking to correct is more narrow than, say, the under eye.

BROW BRUSHES I LIKE:

– Anastasia Beverly Hills 14 Dual Ended Firm Detail

– Anastasia Beverly Hills 7B, 12, 20

– e.l.f. Eyebrow Duo Brush

– BaeBrow Dual Ended Angled Brush

– BaeBrow Brow Groomer and Lash Comb Multitasker

– Bobbi Brown Brow Brush

– Bobbi Brown Eye Definer Brush

– Hannah Martin x Ciaté Brow Brush

– Hannah Martin x Ciaté Spool

– Tweezerman Dual Ended Angled Brow Brush

– Zoeva 322 Brow Line Brush

– NYX Professional Makeup Pro Dual Brow Brush

– Benefit Dual Ended Angled Eyebrow Brush

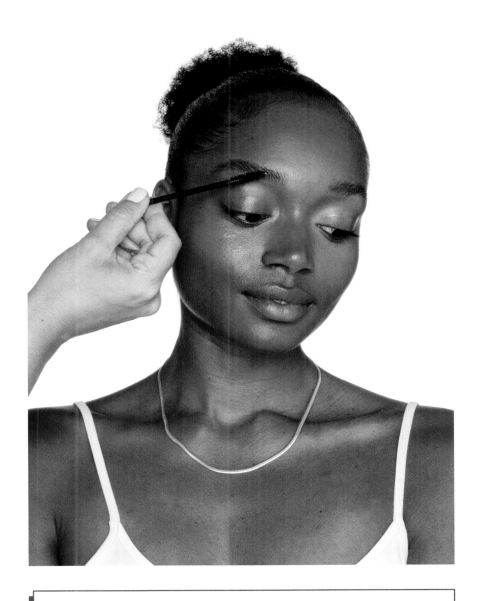

PRACTICE STROKES

I always practise a few strokes on the back of my hand so that I know how it's going to look once I take the brush to my brows. If you don't do this, you run the risk of being too heavy-handed and creating an area of dense pigment in the brows, which can be annoying to try to correct.

MY POPULAR MAKEUP LOOKS

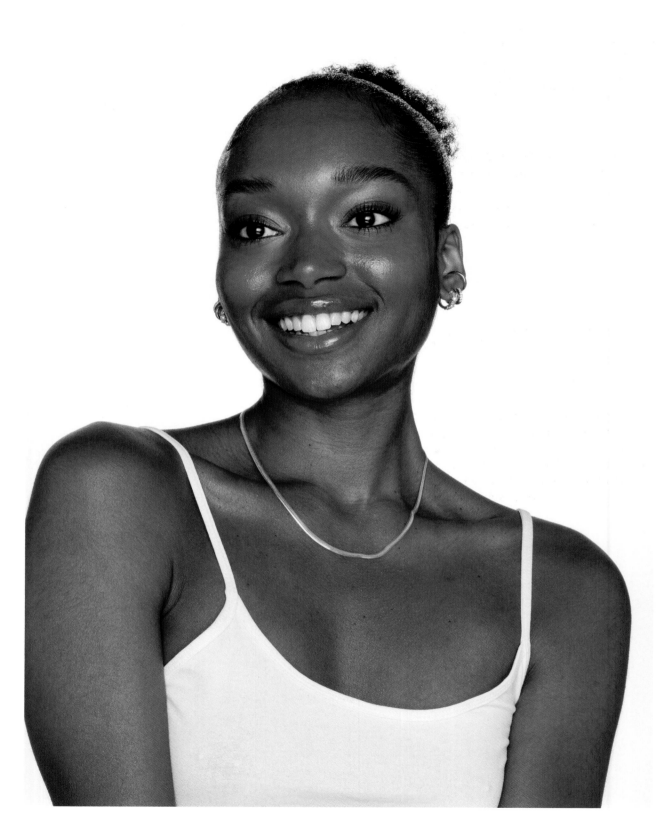

MY POPULAR MAKEUP LOOKS

There are a few looks that I'm asked to create time and time again, so I thought I'd share my tips here. I'd love to know if any of you try to recreate them so, if you do, be sure to share them on social media and tag #hannahmartinmasterclass or #hannahmartinmademedoit!

No-makeup Makeup

Yes, it's a thing! People like to wear makeup to appear as if they're not wearing any makeup. It might sound like it defeats the point, but it enables you to feel polished and pulled together without looking 'made-up'. It's not rocket science, clearly, but it's amazing how many struggle to know how to pare down their makeup, so I hope this helps. As always, it's key to start with clean, cleansed skin.

I used:

- Anastasia BH concealer 21 & 22
- Weleda Skin Food lip balm
- MAC Big Boost fibre gel in onyx
- Clinique High Impact Mascara
- Jones Road in royal plum blush

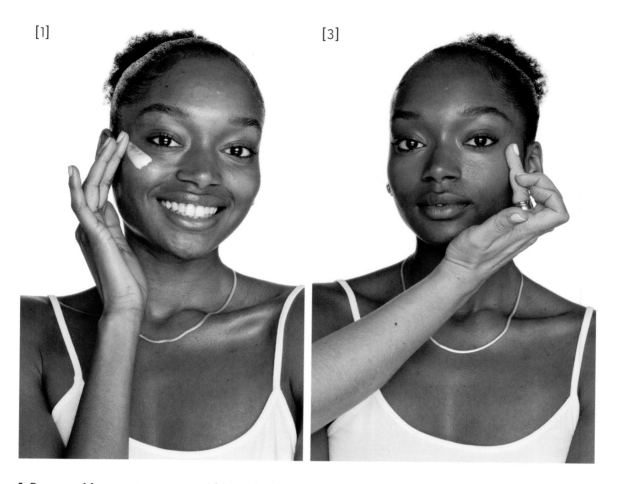

[1]

[3]

1 Do your **skincare** steps as usual (do go back to the skincare section on pages 16–39 if you need reminding about what products to use), and be sure to focus on really hydrating the skin, as a natural glow is key.

2 With a look like this, where the aim is to use as little makeup as possible, it is a good idea to spend a moment **massaging** your skin to help increase circulation and get the blood flowing.

Run the knuckles of your fore and middle fingers along your jawline and either side of your cheekbones, or do the same motion with a roller. Pull in an upward motion to encourage lymphatic drainage, which is particularly

helpful when you are tired, had a lot of salt the night before and your face is puffy.

Apply some pressure under your eyes and sweep your middle finger from either side of the nose, under the eyes and up to the temples.

Smooth above the brows, pressing from the centre of the brows along the brow bone and down towards the temples, your hands mirroring each other at all times.

QUICK TIP:
If you feel any tension in your shoulders, try pinching along the length of your brow . . . it does wonders for releasing tight shoulders! I've

[4]

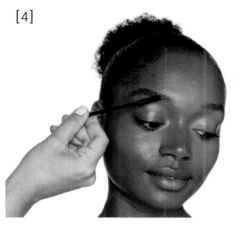

[5]

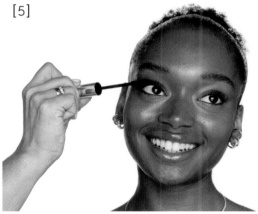

[6]

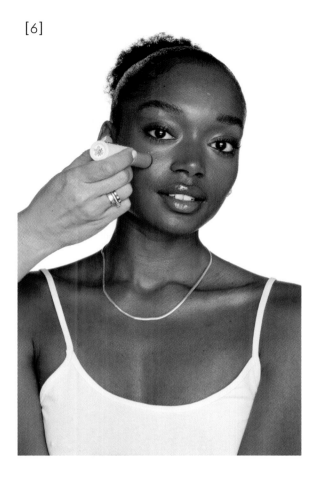

learnt if it's particularly tender in a certain area, it's a good idea to gently pinch and massage that area – there's clearly something tight there.

If you need more help, do watch renowned facialist Nichola Joss's facial massage videos on her Instagram page (@nicholajoss).

3 Once you're familiar with these massage techniques, it's time for a little **concealer** application. Unlike a full makeup look, complete evenness isn't the aim here – it's simply the goal to disguise any redness or blemish that might be grabbing your attention. I usually focus under the eyes and around the nose and chin.

4 It's nice to make the brows look groomed but not overdone, so a slick of **clear brow gel** to hold the hairs in place and slightly define the hairs is perfect, but of course do fill in any gaps that worry you.

5 I tend not to apply mascara for no-makeup makeup looks as it can be obvious, so a simple curl of the lashes will do or, if that feels too 'naked' to you, then do try using a **brown mascara** for a less intense finish.

6 For finishing touches, a dab of **lip balm** on the lips and a touch of a **cream blush** on the cheeks and you're done.

Male Grooming

Whilst everything I've written in this book is applicable to all genders – that's the joy of makeup, it is for anyone and everyone who wants to wear it – more and more I find guys (and women on behalf of men) asking me what little bits of makeup they can use to make themselves feel a bit more put together.

Thankfully, with the emergence of men's skincare and makeup brands, as well as celebrities and influencers openly using and discussing the skincare and makeup they use, guys wearing makeup is no longer seen as taboo. Of course, men can wear makeup traditionally marketed towards women but for some, having skincare and makeup packaged in something specifically targeted to them can help them overcome their nervousness of trying something new.

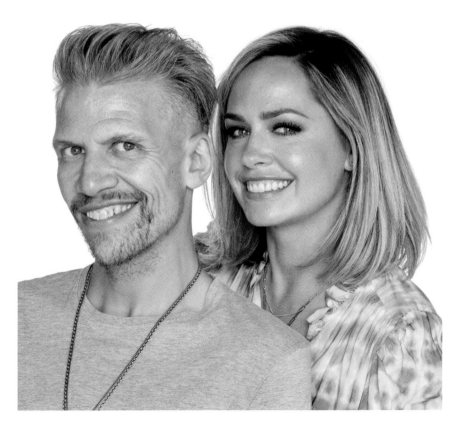

I did a wedding (many years ago now) where the father of the groom was a well-known children's TV personality and I believe he and the groomsmen enjoyed a rather late night before the wedding, so I was summoned from the bridal suite to go and help the lads look a bit more human! Off I scampered (I hadn't factored in any time for male grooming, but I have ever since!) with my moisturiser, concealer palette, bronzing gel and lip balm to revitalise their tired faces before the ceremony. I've since lost count of the times I've been asked to conceal blemishes and tone down redness and mattify a male member of a bridal party.

Side bar: From experience lots of grooms treat themselves to a hot towel shave the morning of their wedding. This is often for the first time and it's key to note that whilst it's a lovely experience sometimes these procedures can leave the skin a little red and often a bit shiny. Neither is a problem but just be aware that this could be the case and your skin might look a bit different to your norm.

My tips for male grooming for those simply wanting to look a little fresher are:

1 Moisturise – Makeup sits better on moisturised skin. Which moisturiser you use depends on your skin type but I usually go for something light like Kiehl's Ultra Facial Cream (my husband likes their Facial Fuel Energising Moisture Treatment For Men) or Clinique Dramatically Different Moisturising Lotion (they also make one targeted to men called Clinique For Men Moisturising Lotion, which feels almost exactly the same).

2 Conceal – Concealing dark circles under the eyes and blemishes can truly transform any complexion. The brighter your under-eye concealer the more obvious it will be, so for something subtle choose a shade that matches your skin tone. The same can be said for a concealer – stick to something the same shade as your face and with a matte finish so that you're not highlighting your spots. Simply apply the concealer where needed and either dab into place with your finger or stipple with a concealer brush. Something like L'Oréal Infallible More Than Concealer or Nars Radiant Creamy Concealer are excellent.

3 Bronze – The ultimate skin revitaliser! Matte powders are brilliant but if you want your makeup to be undetectable then gels are even better. Apply to the top of the forehead, top of the cheeks and place a touch on the nose to add a bit of warmth to the skin. Tom Ford Beauty make an excellent men's gel bronzer as does Clinique, which is very similar.

4 Mattify – There are a number of ways in which you can mattify your skin. A mattifying primer like NYX Shine Killer by War Paint for men; blotting papers like Rodial's Glass Paper or Clean and Clear Oil Control Film or indeed a powder-translucent like Revolution Man Mattifying Powder or Beauty Pie One Powder Wonder.

5 Lip Balm – Keep dry or chapped lips at bay with something like Burt's Bees Moisturising Lip Balm or Le Labo Lip Balm. Neither are too shiny.

6 Eyelash Curler and Brow Groomer – Curling lashes can make all the difference to making eyes look bigger and brighter. I highly recommend both Shiseido and Tweezerman curlers. Tweezerman also make a vast array of brow grooming utensils, but a simple spoolie wand can be excellent for brushing brows into place. A pair of tweezers is essential for plucking unruly brows, or in my husband's case, long curly ones!

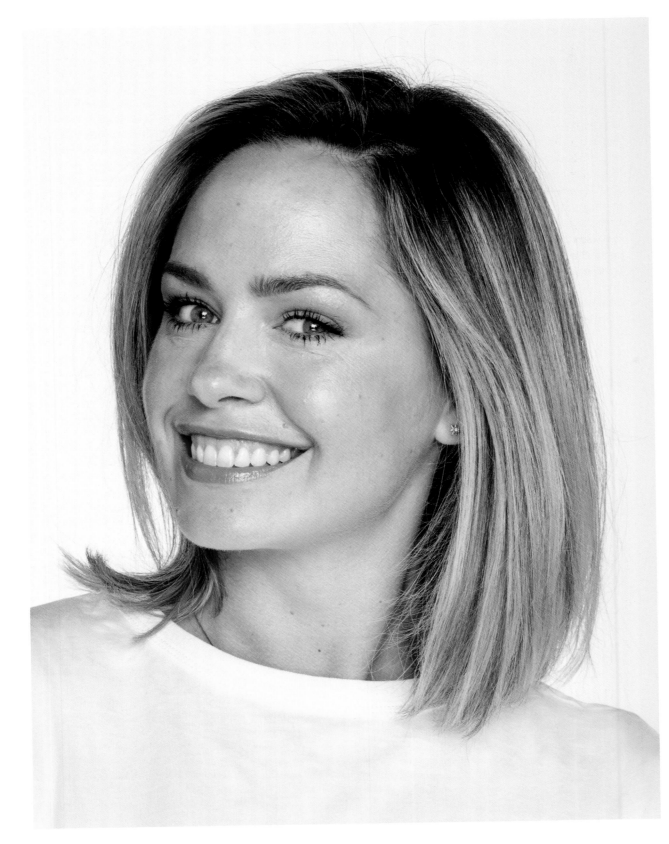

5-Minute Makeup

Time can be a barrier to people applying their makeup. If you don't know a quick routine or your makeup bag is overflowing with lots of products (old and new), then it can all feel a little overwhelming, especially if you're already feeling rushed. That's why I advocate having a separate makeup bag that holds just a few essentials for your day-to-day or for when you find yourself tearing around in a hurry. You can just grab the bag and know you have everything you need for a speedy makeup that could actually really positively impact your day. I know many don't see the power of makeup like I do, but I know that on those most stressful of mornings when I'm getting the kids up and ready for school whilst packing my kit, reading my briefs, checking in on emails … this always makes me feel that little bit brighter. That doesn't mean to say I manage it every day, in fact it's rare that I ever do the school run in makeup!

A note: When we rush it can be tempting to skip skincare, but skincare is always the priority. If you ditch the moisturiser, your foundation will look dry and patchy very quickly. Do please take 20 seconds out of the 5 minutes to apply moisturiser/SPF. The look pictured took less than 5 minutes to film!

I recommend:

- **Moisturiser/SPF**
- **Tinted moisturiser**
- **Concealer**
- **Bronzer**
- **Brow gel**
- **Mascara**
- **Lipstick**

Note: If you have oily skin oil-free tinted moisturiser may be more suitable for you. You can always add powder and setting spray if you want to lock your speedy makeup in place.

I used:

- **La Roche-Posay SFP 50**
- **Code 8 Radiate W20**
- **Urban Decay concealer Stay Naked in 40NN**
- **Huda Beauty Tantour Light**
- **Anastasia Beverly Hills lipstick in dusty rose**
- **Huda Beauty full 'n' Fluffy light brown**
- **MAC Stack mascara in black**

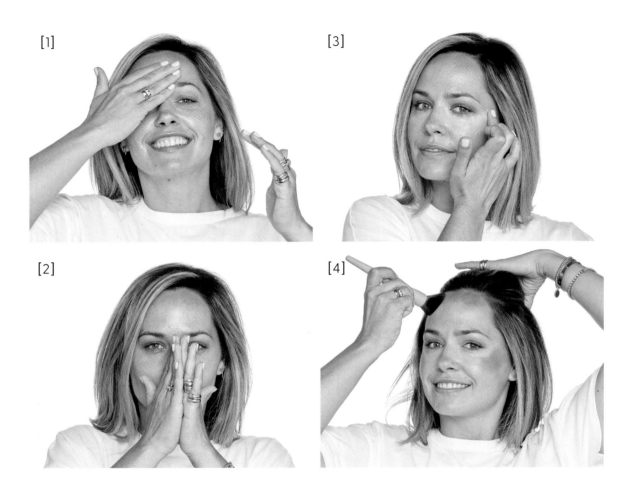

[1]

[2]

[3]

[4]

1 I tend to buy a combination moisturiser/ SPF as many specific facial SPFs do contain excellent moisturisers, for example La Roche-Posay Anthelios Age Correct. This is an SPF 50 face cream that also contains your essentials like hyaluronic acid to moisturise, niacinamide to brighten and lots of antioxidants to protect the skin from damaging free radicals.

2 Follow that with a tinted moisturiser. I love these for speedy makeup as their sheer nature is simply quicker and easier to apply than a more pigmented foundation that may require a bit more care and diligence. Tinted moisturisers are also more emollient, which can be helpful for those days when you don't have time for

an indulgent skincare routine. Just squeeze a large pea-size amount on your fingertips, blend between both hands, then massage into the skin, starting at the nose and blending across the cheek, then sweep the excess over the forehead and take a few seconds to perfect. I find massaging with both hands is much quicker.

3 Apply concealer direct to the skin. Place under the eye and any other area that you want a little extra coverage, usually around the nose, chin and possibly at the front of the cheeks. Then use your fingers or a brush to blend in the concealer. If you have oily hands a synthetic foundation buffing brush will be the perfect tool for this base-perfecting step.

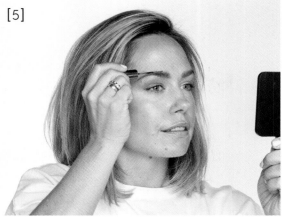

[5]

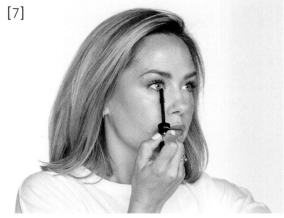

[7]

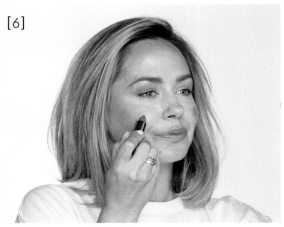

[6]

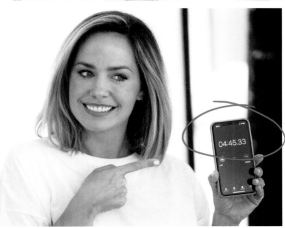

4 Use bronzer powder and a large powder or bronzer brush to sweep the bronzer on the higher points of your face. This includes the forehead (if you're forehead is really narrow then omit this step), top of the cheeks, jawline and neck. Sweep any excess across the bridge of your nose and through the crease of the eye. Four seconds and you have an eye look!

5 I swear by tinted brow gels. I suggest looking for ones with delicate applicators, simply because you'll have more control over a small head than a big spoolie, which can feel a little clumsy. Simply brush through your brows following the direction of the growth of the hairs to add colour, volume and hold the hairs

in place. If your brows are sparse then brush against the direction of the growth and press the spool wand onto the skin to transfer the gel.

6 Apply your lipstick to your lips and also dab some onto the apple of your cheeks and blend out with either a brush or your fingers.

7 Then all that's left is a bit of mascara. A quick curl should only take a few seconds so I highly recommend not skipping this part, it will make a huge difference. For more impact for those rushed days try a more volumising formula so you don't need to layer too much for impact.

Online Makeup

In recent years many of us have found ourselves staring at our colleagues, friends, family and ourselves through the formatively somewhat unfamiliar (but now totally normal) medium that is the virtual meeting place.

Zoom and Microsoft meetings are the new norm, but for many, the sudden shift from maybe only catching sight of their reflection a handful of times a day to staring at themselves on screen all day has been confronting and at times uncomfortable.

> *Laptop cameras aren't necessarily the most flattering, but the placement of the camera will significantly impact how you appear on screen.*

You may not care one bit about how you look (which I applaud) but for those that wish to know, here are my top tips for looking your best online:

- **Sit in front of natural light.** If the window is behind or to the side of you, then your face will appear shadowy and dark. Sit facing the window to make the most of the natural light. If you don't have a window, then a source of light in front of you will help. In my current home I work up in the loft which has sky lights, so I have lights set up behind my tripod to ensure my face isn't shadowed and the makeup is clear in all my videos. I'm not suggesting everyone needs to invest in a fancy lighting system, but there are many simple lighting solutions available: from small clip-on lights that you can attach to the top of your laptop or phone, to tabletop ring-lights you can place on your desk.

- **Raise your laptop or phone** so that the camera is in your eyeline and at head hight. If your device is placed on your desk and you are looking down into the camera, not only will your head be tilted into shadows but the angle of your face is not ideal. You should be able to look straight ahead with your chin raised. You can buy desktop stands, but I simply place my laptop on a stack of books.

If you are wanting to look at your absolute best online, there are five key makeup items, similar to my 5-minute makeup routine (see page 228), that can help you feel camera ready:

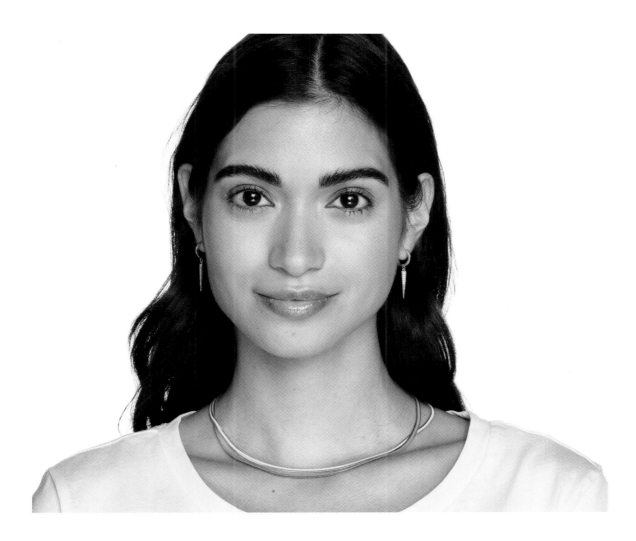

1 Concealer – A little brightening under the eyes can help your eyes look clearer on camera by removing any shadow beneath them. This is especially true for those wearing glasses. Use the same concealer to tone down any redness in the skin.

2 Mascara – Volumised, lifted and lengthened lashes will make your eyes a focal point, framing them and helping to open the eyes. It is key, though, that you curl your lashes beforehand as it will make all the difference in helping you create that lifted, fanned look.

3 Brows – A little definition through the brows will help to add structure to your face and further frame your eyes, which will help when trying to 'connect' with others through a screen.

4 Blush – A bit of colour on the apples of your cheeks can help you look fresh and healthy.

5 Lip Balm – A hydrated lip looks good and feels good. By all means wear your favourite lip colour, but if in doubt reach for something that will moisturise and add a little sheen, as matte lips can look flat on camera.

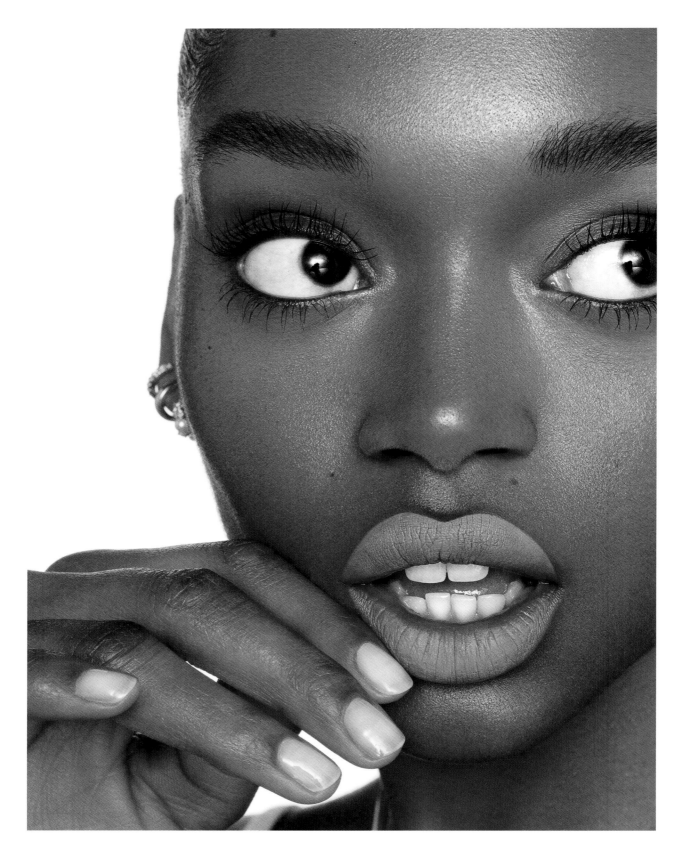

Bold Lips

I am a self-confessed lipstick addict, I really am. I own more than I should and my husband despairs whenever another lipstick purchase arrives, but I just love how lipstick makes me feel.

I'm always experimenting with different shades and textures but the biggest discovery came to me a few years ago when I realised the only thing holding me back from wearing certain lipstick colours was what I thought others would think of me. Does that resonate with any of you? I worried that people would think I was attention-seeking if I wore a bold colour or a sparkly gloss, so for years I really played down my lipstick colour choice.

I think a lot of us 'fear' lipstick colours and worry more about the perception of ourselves in the bold lip colour than fulfilling our desire to give the bolder colours a go. I now have a much freer relationship with lipstick. Since I started to care less about what people think, I've discovered immense joy in wearing bold lipsticks.

Lipstick isn't for everyone, but it's easy to take off and change and it doesn't last forever, so if you fancy donning a bright orange, then go for it! I prefer to keep the rest of the makeup pared down so the lip colour does all the talking. That's not to say that you can't do it all – full base, big eyes and a bold lip – you absolutely can!

I've set out here my favourite combination for a bold lip look but, of course, this is just a suggestion and totally open to interpretation.

I used:

- **Fresh lip scrub**
- **Bobbi Brown lip balm**
- **Confession Ultra Slim High Intensity Refillable Lipstick Red 0**
- **Charlotte Tilbury lip pencil in Kiss 'N' Tell**

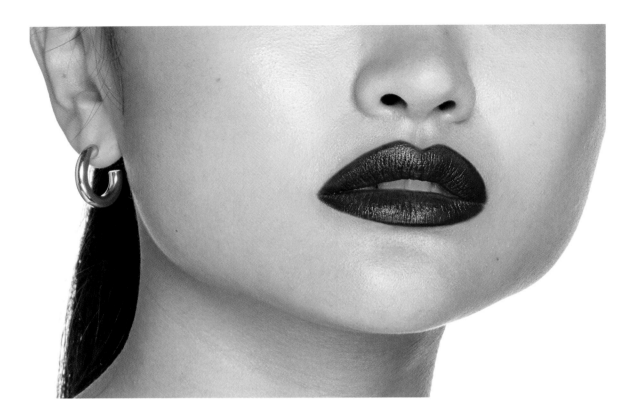

COLOUR

Red is a bold colour and it works across all skin tones, but I also like to make a statement with oranges, fuchsia pinks, deep berry and plums – and the ultimate in bold … black. Yes, I said black – it's not everyone's cup of tea, but do you remember the image of Rihanna when her brand **Fenty** launched the **Stunna Lip Paint** in **Uninvited**? I loved it – such a powerful look – and lots of brands swiftly followed suit on the back of its success.

Black lips are no longer synonymous with gothic-style makeup and witches, with many fashion houses choosing the shade for their fashion week runways and celebrities for glamorous red-carpet moments. If black is a step too far for you, then Rihanna's **Underdawg** is a gorgeous super-deep red alternative – think **Rouge Noir** but for lips.

I will just caveat here that if you rarely wear lipstick, any colour will feel bold initially. So, don't panic if a mid-pink feels bold, that's totally ok and I hold space for you too. This is just a section where I'm discussing deeper, brighter, densely pigmented lip colours and how to wear them. So, back to application.

1 When you're wanting to make a statement with a stronger lip colour, it's a good idea to create a base that neutralises any redness in the skin. I prefer this so that the palette is even, allowing the lipstick to be the focus. I'd suggest a **medium coverage base makeup** and **concealer**.

2 Whilst I'm a huge fan of blue-based pink blusher, I won't use pink blush when creating a bold lip as it can steal focus away from the lipstick. I prefer a more minimalist look and neutral colour palette. I do add **bronzer**, as long as it's a bronzer that suits your skin tone but is not overly done, with just enough warmth that you don't look pale. I'd suggest a neutral blush shade: think **MAC Melba** for fairer skins and **MAC Film Noir** for black skin, which works well on fair to deep black and brown skins.

3 A defined brow is a good idea when wearing a bold lip. A bit like with a smokey eye, I feel brows need to match the intensity of your focus area. It makes sense to fill in your brows with a touch more intensity than usual. If you don't, your brows can look a little light and insipid next to the lip.

4 When it comes to **eye makeup** with a bold lip, again, I teach that less is more. Of course, there is no rule that says you must not have dark eyes and dark lips, but I like the lips to be the focus, so I tend to keep the eyes bare.

For all skin tones, you can't go wrong with matte neutral tones not dissimilar to the natural colour of the skin on the lids. I suggest shadow as it absorbs any natural oil on the lids and creates a more polished finish.

On Caucasian skin, I adore a light, slightly frosted shade – a light champagne or cold silver – all over, with a slightly warmer crease colour (a very pale muted peach is lovely, as is

a pale mushroom), then a decent bit of eyeliner pushed right in between the lashes as tight lining to define the eyes. Alternatively, a bold lip with a sheer eye can look very sexy and more feline if you fill in the waterline on the top and lower lid.

Tight lining:
We call applying the eyeliner in between the lashes 'tight lining', although I think even MUAs have varying ideas about what this means. My understanding is that this is the practice of getting liner just in between the lashes and not on the actual waterline. I avoid the waterline if I'm not going to fill the entirety of it. This is because if the pencil liner gets on to the waterline, it can transfer to the lower line and you're left with a slightly murky look. If you focus just between the lashes, you'll get the intensity and definition that helps your lashes look fuller but without the transfer.

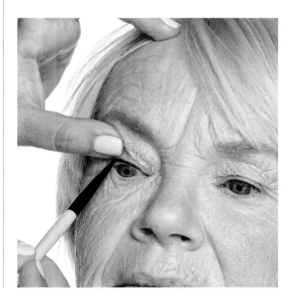

On brown and black skin, I think it can be impactful to go sheer and cool with the shadow and do a light wash of a cool silver. Not a bold, intense metallic, but instead something much more subtle – a sparkle maybe, like **Shiseido's Aura Dew in Lunar**. If, however, the cool contrast doesn't appeal to you, then a warm gold has a similar effect.

5 Complete the eye look with lashings of **mascara**. Don't hold back as the shadow here is minimal, so the mascara really is the main feature and, like the brows, the intensity of your mascara should match the intensity of the focus area.

6 When applying your bold lip, it may be helpful to use lip liner first if you're at all concerned about the lip colour application, but may I also suggest you have cotton buds, eye makeup remover and concealer to hand for perfecting your lip edge.

You can get teeny-tiny cotton buds from MyKitCo and Muji and they are so helpful when it comes to tweaking lipstick.

Anchor your hand by resting your little finger on your chin and then slowly but surely start to edge the lips. Keep the pencil in contact with the skin and do very small strokes back and forth, gradually extending to complete the liner. With bold lip colours, I do suggest filling in the entire lip with a lip pencil or at least blending the liner down into the lip a little. This prevents being left with a really dark line around the lip edge as the lipstick wears off.

QUICK TIP
If your liner pencil is cold or hasn't been used in a while, then you may find that the nib has gone a bit hard or has 'oxidised' and not a huge amount of colour is translating onto the skin. If this happens, don't worry, it's easily fixed.

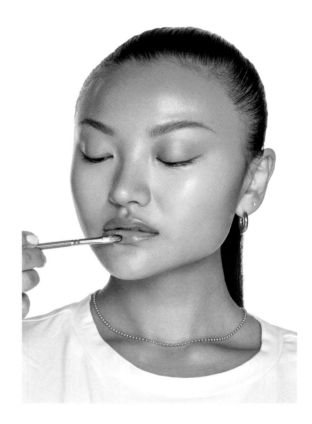

Give the pencil a sharpen and then work it into the back of your hand to warm it up. Don't persevere with a hard nib as you won't get any product on the lip and you may make the lips a bit pink if you press too hard.

7 Once you're happy with the liner, follow on top with the lip colour of your choice. Take it slowly when using a bold colour, as precision is key. If you feel your lipstick bullet is a bit big and you're struggling to have complete control, it can be useful to invest in a lip brush. They're usually slanted flat with curved edges to help hug the contour of your lips.

Again, anchor your hand by placing your little finger on the chin. This just helps to steady your hand, as doing anything completely freehand can be challenging.

[7]

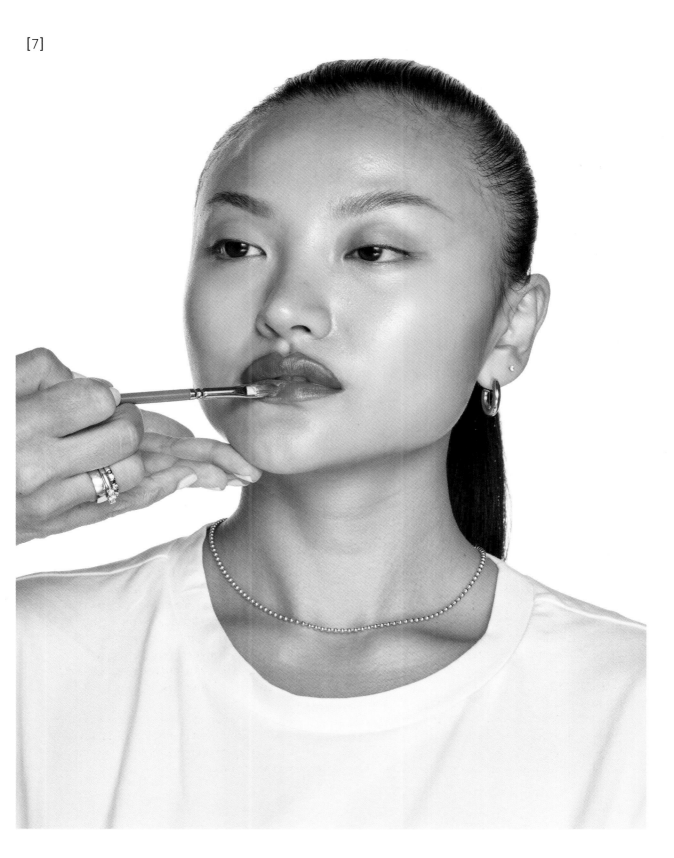

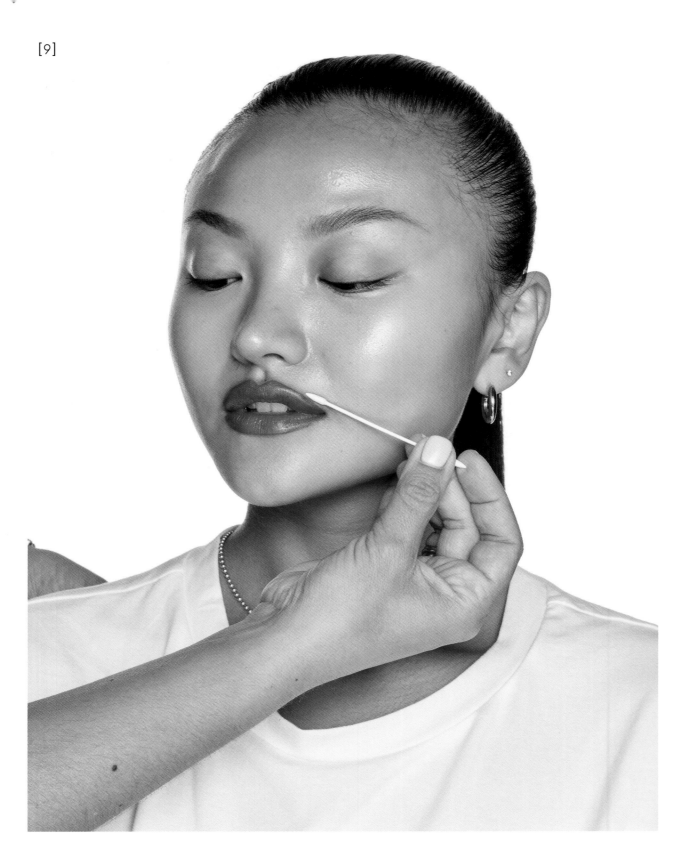

[9]

BLOTTING

Once the colour is applied, it can be a good idea to blot the lipstick with a tissue and reapply. This was one of the very first makeup tips that I ever read and I have read it many, many times since, but it really does work. Un-blotted deep lip colours can feel a bit 'wet', especially if they are more moisturising formulas, so blot the lipstick to take any excess product off that could otherwise end up on the teeth or being smudged.

You can also powder the lipstick if it is a bit moist to help keep it in place better. Dab some translucent powder directly onto the lip or push some powder on a brush through a one-ply tissue.

8 More often than not, I will then go round the lip edge again with the lip pencil to further perfect the contour. I know this sounds like a lot, but there's nothing more irritating than looking back at a beauty shot and the lip edge not being completely perfect . . .

9 If you've neatened the edge with your lip pencil but still fear it's not perfect or if, in fact, you made a little mistake, don't panic, this is where those tiny cotton buds and that bit of eye makeup remover come in handy.

Dip the cotton bud in the remover then firmly pull it under the mistake to remove it. Just be careful about using the same cotton bud to perfect any other areas as it may well have absorbed some of the lip colour. On many occasions I've gone to do another tweak and as I've pulled the cotton bud across the skin, I've left a trail of the colour behind me and given myself yet more to fix! Most annoying.

10 Once you're happy with the shape, you can then apply a bit of concealer around the lip edge to perfect. This may not be necessary but sometimes bold reds can stain the skin a little, so it can be helpful to use a bit of concealer to correct it. Adjust using a minimal amount of product on a very slim, flat concealer or lip brush.

Using Concealer to Perfect Lips

You can use a lighter concealer if you want to make a point of outlining the lips, but I prefer a shade that matches the tone of the skin around the lips so it's less obvious.

One little note to any MUAs reading: whilst concealer is an excellent tool to perfect bold lips, don't allow yourself to become reliant on this technique as it doesn't work with everyone, specifically those with fine, downy hair on their skin, as the concealer will collect in the fine hairs and start to look a little congealed. The concealer then creates texture and the texture creates shadow and thus highlights the hairs, which can make it look like there's more hair than there actually is. I have a lot of hair on my top lip and avoid using too much product otherwise it really exacerbates their appearance.

FINAL TOUCHES

A little splash of highlight can really set off and finish a bold lip look, so do try highlighting a little under the brow bone, in the inner corner of the eyes and even the cupid's bow.

LIP PENCILS

You may have had hard lip pencils in the past, but there are lots available now that are soft and creamy. Do test the intensity of the formula on the back of your hand before going to the lip – it would be a real shame if you pressed too hard and either broke the nib of your liner or simply applied too much product. I like to use a small domed brush like the buffer brush from my collection with Ciaté as its density helps to apply the shadow intensely to the lip. A fluffier brush will create a softer finish.

A BOLD POWDER LIP

A bold powder lip is also a firm favourite, but it's not at all long-wearing. It's exactly what it sounds like: you sweep dark shadows or blush over the lips with a brush.

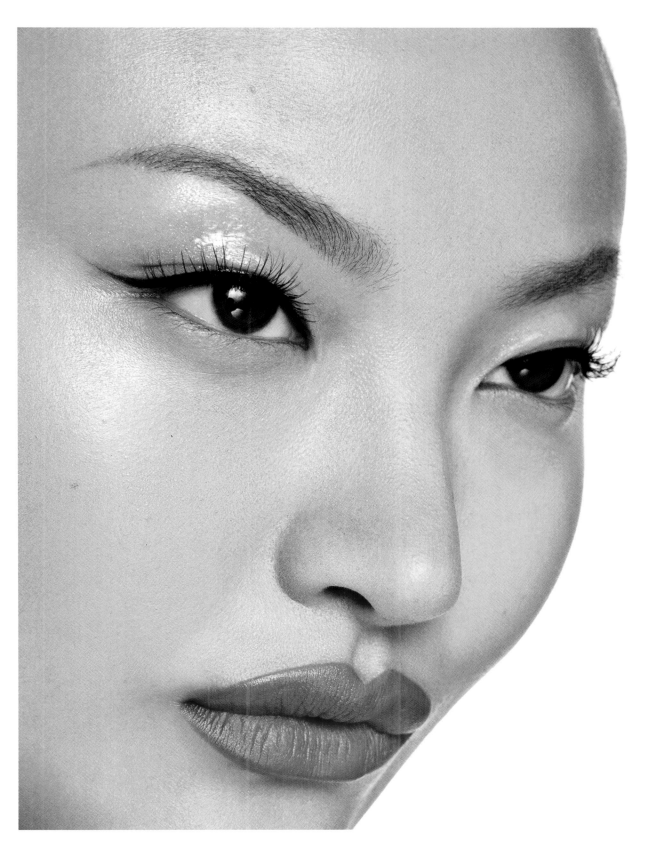

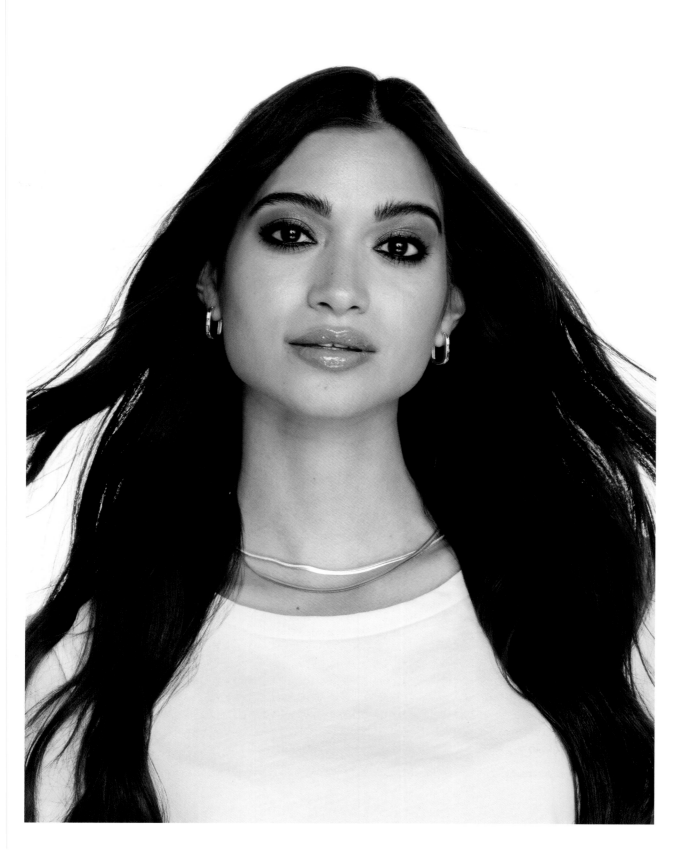

Smokey Eyes

For many years, smokey eyes were the most searched makeup trend on the internet.

In fact, one of my very first makeup looks that I mastered as a young teen was a version of the smokey eye – a dark base with a black sparkly shadow I bought on the high street. I am pretty sure it had something to do with an All Saints music video.

The smokey eye first became popular back in the 1920s when people started copying the makeup they saw in the films. It was all black and white back then, so all shades looked fairly intense on screen. Makeup shades were also limited, so the block colour smokey eye quickly became popular. Although it has evolved over time, the principle is still the same: a single colour smudged all around the eyes that's well blended and diffused with no hard lines.

I was taught years ago the simple principle that our thoughts affect our feelings and our feelings affect our behaviour. If you do your makeup and you think you look good, those positive thoughts will positively affect how you feel and in turn there will be a positive impact on how you behave. I've heard so many times in my adult life that makeup is fickle or for the vain, but as Sali Hughes says, makeup is the simple act of self-care.

I stand by the notion that smokey eyes are so popular because of how it makes the wearer feel. When it comes to applying a smokey eye it's not

I used:

- **Anastasia Beverly Hills brow powder in ebony**
- **Blink Brow Bar in clear eye gloss**
- **Charlotte Tilbury Eyes To Mesmerise in Mona Lisa**
- **Anastasia Beverly Hills Sultry Palette in birch**
- **Delilah black gel**

- **Tweezerman lash curlers**
- **Lancôme Hypnôse Mascara in black**
- **Urban Decay 24/7 eye pencil in black**
- **Anastasia Beverly Hills Sultry in noir - under lash line**

- **Anastasia Beverly Hills sultry in ember - top lid**
- **Bobbi Brown Smokey Quartz sparkle**
- **Nabla Glorious Light Palette**
- **Maybelline Lifter Gloss in ice**

as difficult as it may seem. This look is most synonymous with charcoals, blacks and greys, but browns and bronzes are stunning, too, as are bold colours – I love a lilac smokey eye, for example.

One of the most simple smokey eyes that I teach involves just three items: a **shadow**, a **liner** and a **mascara**. Whilst the exact shade of the shadow is up to you, I will just say that the shadow colour should be deeper than your skin tone for the finish to be effective. Whilst I do love a silvery based smokey eye on black and brown skin, and therefore not deeper than the skin tone, you'll notice that while there may be silver on the moveable part of the lid, the lash lines are usually significantly deeper, often black, to create that deep smokiness required. Without that darker framing with the black it won't really look or feel like a smokey eye.

You can use any texture of shadow you like – matte, shimmer, metallic, sparkle or cream. If you're using a powder shadow and your lids are naturally a bit oily you may want to prime your lid with an eye base. If you do this with concealer or foundation, just be careful that you use the tiniest bit and really blend it out as too much can cause the shadows to crease. I therefore prefer to use primers like the iconic Urban Decay Primer Potion but a long-wear cream shadow in a neutral colour like a MAC paint pot will also work. You can then apply your shadow on top.

If you don't want to use a long-wear cream shadow as a base, although I highly recommend this for locking your look in place, you can prep the lid with a matte shadow in a similar tone to absorb any oil on the lid and give your powder shadows something to blend into, as the shadow can get 'caught' on slightly moist skin. You'll know if this has happened as you may find it hard to blend evenly through the crease, or see little drag marks or general inconsistency in the shadow colour. You can also prep the lids with a very light layer of really well-blended concealer set with powder. If the concealer on the lid is thick or wet it can cause shadows to crease.

IN A HURRY?

I should quickly point out that I can do a smokey eye in under five minutes if I use a long-wear cream shadow stick. I love Bark from Bobbi Brown, Cocoa by NudeStix or Raven by Vieve. Just blend the shade all over the lid and blend out with your finger – it's that easy! Do the same along the lower lash line and finish with mascara. Super simple speedy smokey eyes for when time is of the essence.

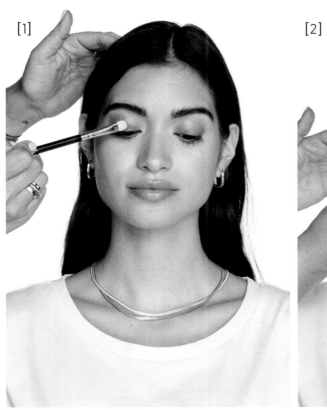

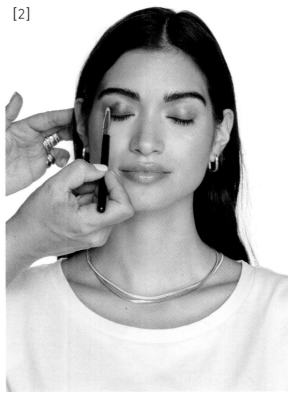

1 When it comes to creating a smokey finish with your shadow, especially when using deeper tones, I suggest using a pressing motion. Dab your eyeshadow brush into your shadow of choice and be sure to tap it into the palm of your hand to push the pigment into the brush. Then, with your eyes open, head back slightly, start gently pressing the side of the brush head into the centre of your eyelid with the brush horizontal and angled out to the side. This might sound odd but trust me when I say this will really help you lay the colour down without it falling. If you hold the brush pointing directly towards you and try to blend with the tip of the brush head there are two areas for error. Your view will be obscured because all you can see is the brush and your hand but also the brush head is likely to hit your eyelashes and cause shadow to fall. Avoid using any

windscreen-wiper motion at this point as there is too much pigment in your brush and you don't yet have the base of your colour on the lid.

2 Start in the centre of the lid and then gradually move to the outer corner of the eye, then into the inner corner. You shouldn't need to reload your brush but if you do be sure to push the powder into the brush head again. Keep dabbing until you build an even layer of colour on the lower lid. When you're happy, turn your brush vertically and start dabbing the brush head into the crease of the eye, gradually dabbing the brush higher through the crease to bring the shadow colour that little bit higher. Reload the brush with pigment if necessary and when you think you have the right intensity of colour through the crease that's when I

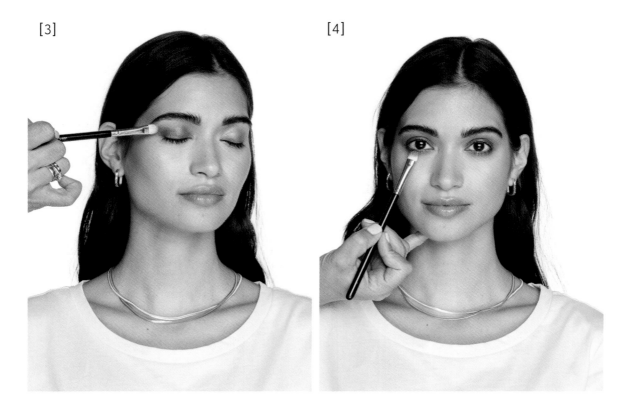

start a bit of the windscreen-wiper motion, sweeping the brush from left to right through the crease of the eye to further blend the shadow, bringing it up onto the brow bone but not all the way up to it. Keep the brush in contact with the skin at all times as this will help your blending.

NOTE:

For those with hooded or downturned eyes, be sure not to bring the colour too far down in the outer corner of the eye – draw an imaginary line from the outer corner of your eye to the end of your brow and no shadow goes past that line – it will just help your eyes look lifted.

3 I love to pull the shadow out a little towards the tail of the brow. It creates a slightly more feline look and prevents your smokey eye from looking too round.

4 Then take the same shadow and brush and smudge it along the lower lash line. Be careful not to overload the brush with shadow, it's easier to start with less and add than it is to blend away too much. Gradually build the colour all along the lash line. I start at the centre and blend out to the outer corner, then along into the inner corner. You can make the lower lash line shadow much deeper than you might expect. If the liner is narrow it can look a little harsh or stark, so don't be afraid to bring the shadow lower than you think you ought to. If you're unsure how far to take the lower lash line shadow, try taking a selfie and seeing how it's translating on camera. If you're using a really dark colour it may help to gently line the lower lash line with your bronzer or another slightly lighter shadow. Just be sure to blend your shadow well in the outer corner so the base line of the shadow looks smooth. If it's

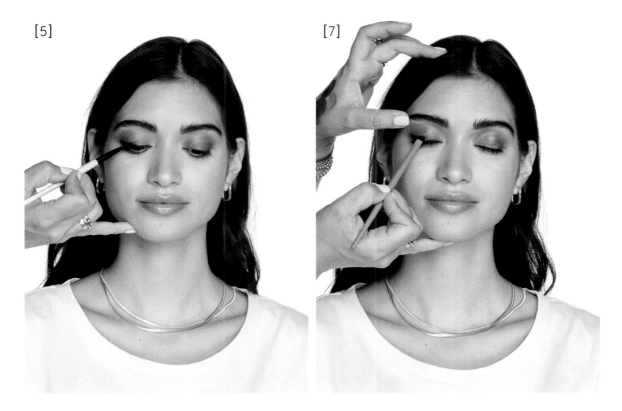

a little uneven, don't panic, you can neaten up the line using a bit of concealer on a flat concealer brush.

5 Now it's time for liner, and in my opinion, more is more! My preference is to use a soft kohl or kajal that you can blend for the ultimate smudgy smokiness. If you want to use a liquid liner, apply your liner and take a shadow the same colour and blend it all over the top edge of the liner – this is known as double lining – so you get all the intensity of the liquid line at the base of the lashes and then the darkest colour bleeds up into the lower lid.

6 If using a kohl or kajal you don't have to be too precise, just etch the liner all along the lash line, being sure to work the liner right in between the lashes as any hint of skin can break up the intensity.

7 Then with a small-headed shadow brush like the Morphe M210, start smudging and buffing the liner out, pulling the colour up the lid. It's key to point out here that you're aiming to smudge the top of the liner. If you start smudging at the base of the liner, at the lash line, you could diffuse the colour. If you're using a longer-lasting eyeliner, be mindful that due to their waterproof formula these pencils are usually not as soft and dry quite quickly, so you don't have much time to blend. Therefore, do one eye at a time and don't hesitate when it comes to smudging, have the brush you're going to use poised and ready to go.

8 To make a smokey eye really intense, I love to tight line the top lash line and fill in the waterline too, it just cancels out that flesh colour. Adding liner to the lower waterline adds a bit of drama too. To make sure the lower liner

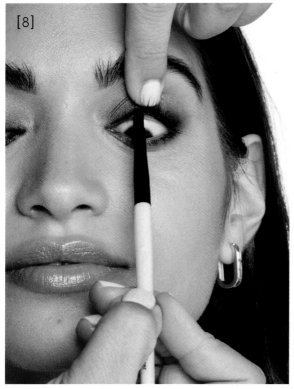

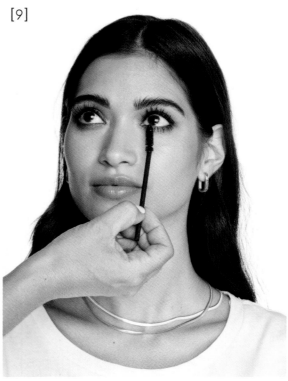

is as intense as possible, be sure to shade every bit of skin between the lashes. Once I've taken the liner along the waterline, under the lashes and blended, I often take a dark shadow in a slim, small-headed brush and push the shadow into the lower lashes from above the lash line, to cover any skin that might be showing.

9 I use lots of mascara on this look. For the mascara to be seen you must curl the lashes first and then apply a few coats of your favourite volumising mascara. Like brows, the intensity of your mascara needs to match that of the shadow, so if you've done a super dark eye then you need big lashes, so take your time. Push the wand of your mascara into the base of your lashes then start to drag the wand slowly through the lashes. Do this repeatedly along your entire lash line, being sure to pull straight up towards your brows in the centre.

Then pull the inner lashes in towards your nose and the lashes in the outer corner towards the tip of your brow for the fullest, most fanned-out effect. I always do the lower lashes too. I turn the wand vertically to tease the lower lashes bit by bit – I find this technique prevents me from getting mascara on the skin blow the lashes. If you find your mascara smudges on the lower lashes then do try a waterproof or tubing formula to prevent this and make sure your concealer under the eye is totally dry before application.

There's lots more you can do to tweak a smokey eye – add a lighter shade to the inner corner of the eye, press a little sparkle into the centre of the lid, highlight the brow bone with a little highlighter – the possibilities are endless.

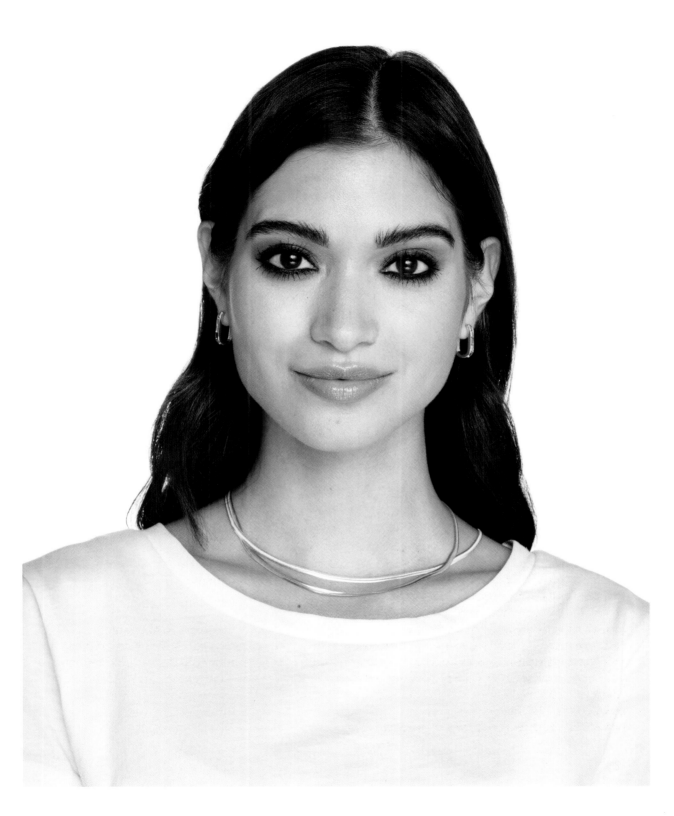

Mature Skin

I've always been a firm believer that makeup is something to be enjoyed. I don't buy into the idea that one should stop enjoying makeup when one hits a certain age. However, I do recognise that certain textures and finishes suit mature skin better than others and that some techniques and styles can date your look.

I say that because it's common to meet with women who replicate the makeup style they adopted in their youth and continue it throughout their adult life. This is of course absolutely fine – if you love it and it makes you feel good then wear it – but it's worth noting that as well as fashions changing over time, so do your colouring and features. I'm particularly thinking of black eyeliner, which can become overpowering and negate its purpose. Instead, you could define an eye with a softer colour and not overpower the eyes.

Mature skin will also benefit from a more hydrated, glowing base. Completely matte textures can exacerbate the appearance of fine lines so I suggest lightweight, hydrating bases to give the skin a more radiant, modern appearance. Then layer with cream colour on top – cream bronzer and cream blush, specifically.

I used:

- MAC Face & Body in N3
- Bobbi Brown Light Bisque corrector
- Bobbi Brown Concealer in sand
- Mehron cream bronzer/ contour in medium 4
- Clé de Peau Beauté blush cream 2
- Anastasia Beverly Hills brow powder in ash
- Charlotte Tilbury Eyes to Mesmerise in champagne
- Delilah black gel for tight line
- Delilah brown gel for lash line
- Charlotte Tilbury Pillow Talk palette in crease
- Tweezerman lash curlers
- L'Oréal Paradise
- Rimmel lip liner in Call me Crazy
- Ciaté in lychee & açai conditioning lip oil

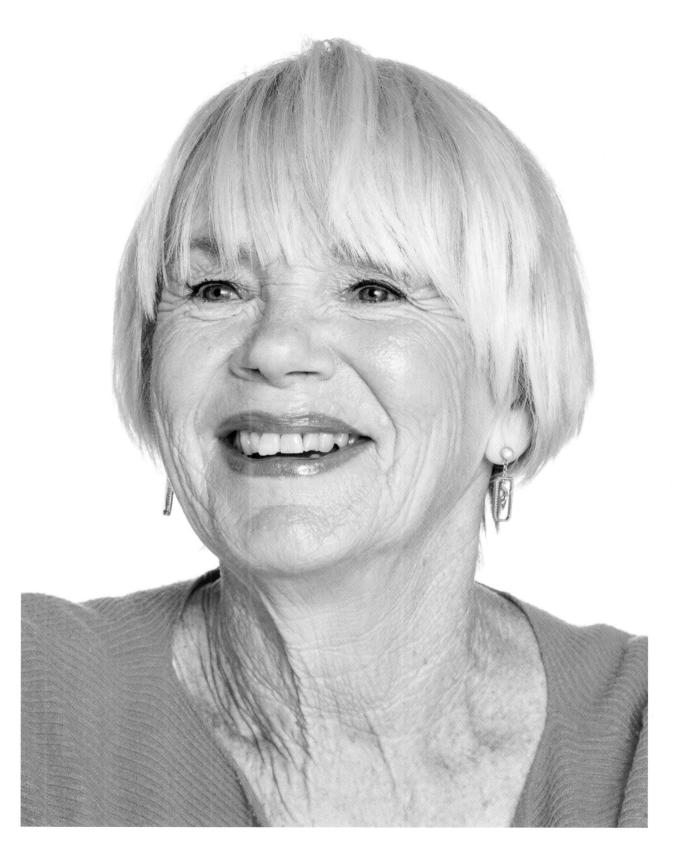

1   Prep the skin with hydrating skincare (essence, serum, eye cream, face cream, SPF).

2   Even the skin tone with a lightweight base, such as Estée Lauder Futurist Hydra Rescue. Be wary of too much powder as this may dull the glow of the base, and it's not entirely necessary unless your skin is on the oily side.

3   Brighten the under eyes with corrector (if needed) and hydrating concealer, such as IT Cosmetics Bye Bye Under Eye.

4   Warm the edges of the face with a cream bronzer, such as Fenty Cream Bronzer.

5   Add a pop of colour to the apple of the cheeks with a cream blush, such as Bobbi Brown Pale Pink Pot Rouge.

6   Define the brows with a brow powder, such as Anastasia Beverly Hills Brow Powders and set in place with a brow gel. If your brows have lost their colour, then try a tinted brow gel like the Benefit Gimme Brow Gel.

7   Sweep a wash of shadow all over the lid and through the crease of the eye. I use long-wear cream shadows as they adhere well and don't move, which is helpful on more delicate lids.

8   Define the eye with a little liner right into the root of the lashes. I love to buff and smudge the liner for a softer finish.

9   Curl the lashes and apply a few coats of mascara so that they are very visible. While some like a brown mascara, I feel black defines lashes the best.

10 Finish with creamy lipstick to ensure lips look their fullest. If you feel you've lost a little definition or volume to the lip, do line them first with a lip pencil, being sure to go to the furthest extent of the lip edge and even slightly over it if you want to increase the appearance. A gloss on top of your lipstick will add to the effect.

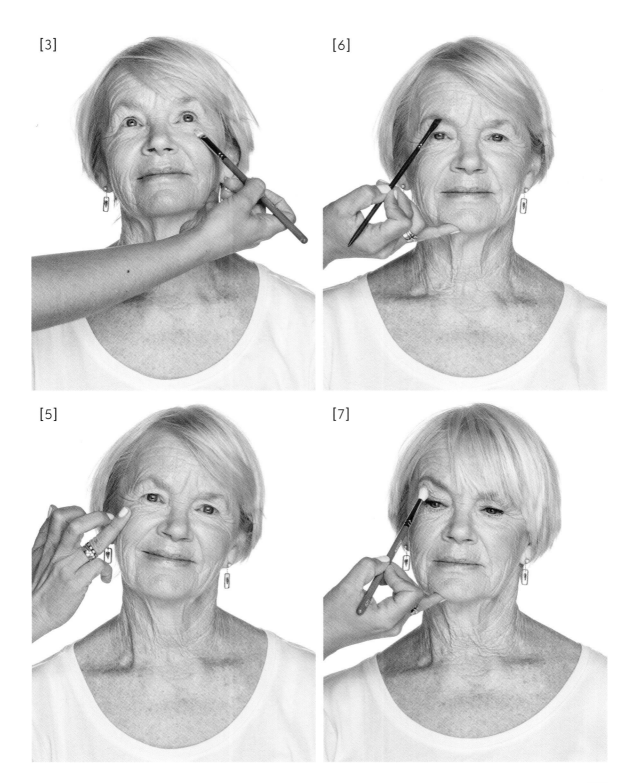

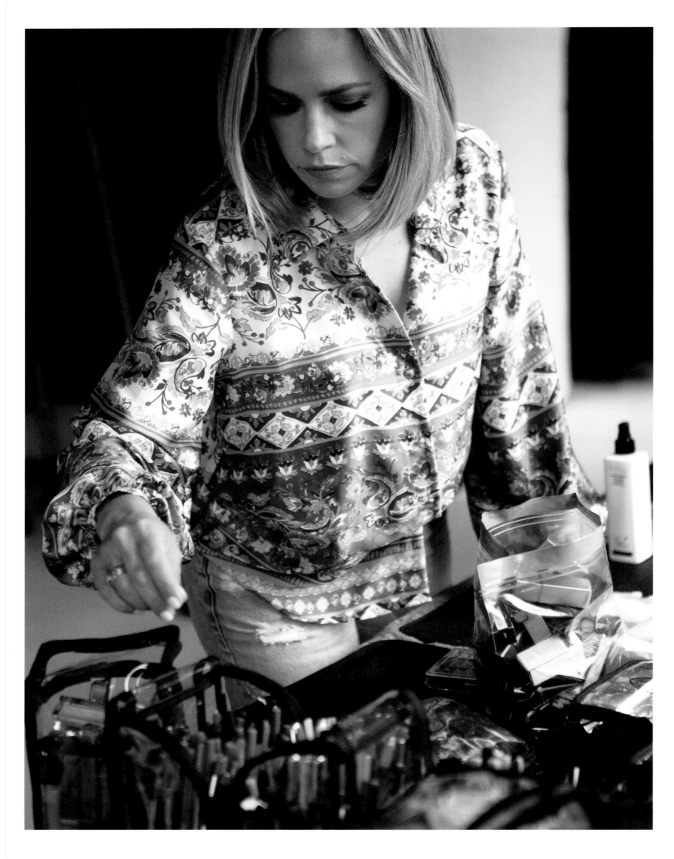

Long-wear/Waterproof Makeup

Long-wear makeup is totally different to beauty shoot makeup. Shoot makeup doesn't need to last, it just needs to look good in the moment for the photographer to get the shot. Sadly we're not always lit by professionals or have makeup artists on hand for touch ups every few minutes, so some of the gorgeous looks we see in glossy magazines or online don't translate brilliantly when it comes to longevity. But, thankfully, there are lots of products out there that can withstand a trip to the gym, a swim in the sea, high humidity or an 18-hour day!

You don't have to use all these products mentioned, as long-wear makeup doesn't have to be full makeup. A few simple formula tweaks and you really can create plenty of looks that don't smudge at all.

1 If longer wear is important to you then you need to start taking this into consideration at the very first step of your routine – your skincare. Look for products that don't contain oil and stick to water-based serums and moisturisers like Vichy Mineral 89 Hyaluronic Acid Serum and follow with something like Kiehl's Ultra Facial Oil-Free Gel Cream. The same goes when choosing your SPF and foundation. There are many to choose from, but I do love Eucerin Oil Control Sun Gel-Cream SPF 50 for oily skin.

2 There are plenty of foundation options available but the bareMinerals Complexion Rescue foundation stick is water-based, gorgeous and in no way heavy. For fuller coverage, pick oil-free formulas like Charlotte Tilbury's Airbrush Flawless Foundation and Bobbi Brown Skin Long-Wear Weightless. Estée Lauder's Double Wear Foundation is a full coverage foundation but you can apply just a little for a more sheer application, and it has such a loyal fanbase because it really doesn't move.

3 Setting with powder is essential for long-wearing makeup but again, look for one that is oil free, as not all are. A few favourites are Clinique Stay Matte oil-free powder and Charlotte Tilbury's Airbrush Flawless Finish Powder. It is best to use powder-based blush as it lasts better than creams.

4 For brows there are lots of long-wear brow pencils and pomades available – you really don't need to look further than Anastasia Beverly Hills for everything you could need. I do recommend you avoid powder

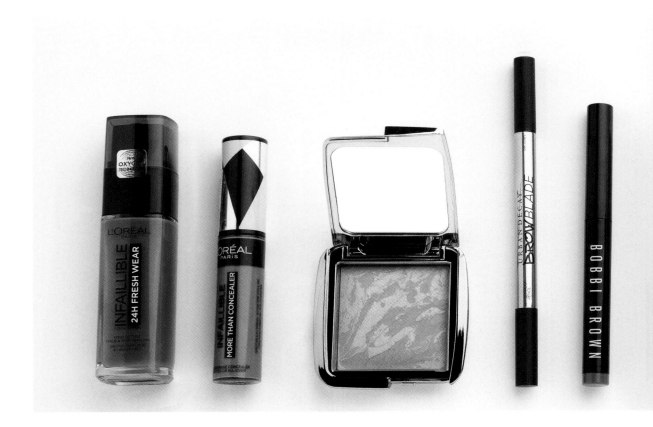

on the brows, which can move as you sweat, whereas a waterproof pomade won't budge.

5 When it comes to eye makeup I'd always recommend long-wear cream shadows. Long gone are the days of tubes of cream containing pigment that didn't even last five minutes on the skin without creasing. Now there are multiple liquid formulas like Huda Beauty's Matte and Metal Melted Shadows – I wore their Diamond Drip shadow when I ran the London Marathon and it DID NOT MOVE! You can also find excellent waterproof eyeliners, such as Urban Decay 24/7 which is a glide on pencil that is smooth on application and doesn't smudge (they are therefore my go-to for brides).

6 Waterproof or tubing mascara is best for long-wear. Unfortunately, not all waterproof mascaras are created equal so be sure to look up reviews before you make your purchase. Some of the best include Bobbi Brown No Smudge, Clinique High Impact Waterproof and Huda Legit Lashes Waterproof Topcoat. You will need to also purchase a waterproof makeup remover like Lancôme Bi-Facil as most cleansers will struggle to lift the makeup off! If the removal process puts you off, then a tubing

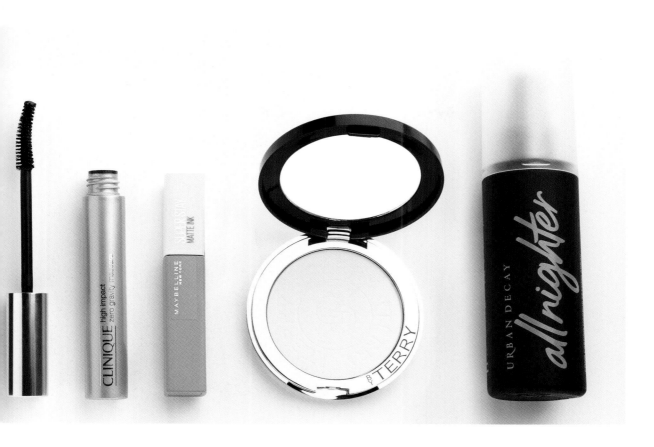

mascara is a great alternative. The polymers wrap themselves around the lashes and create little 'tubes' of coating that only come off when teased with warm water. It makes removal really easy and doesn't break or pull your lashes, there are great options by Trish McEvoy, Hourglass Unlocked and Victoria Beckham.

7 Liquid lipsticks tend to be the most long-wearing. Until recently the only real option for waterproof lipstick was Max Factor Lipfinity, which is still one of the very best smudge-resistant lipsticks on the market, but admittedly it does dry over time, which is why it comes with a gloss to revive it. Recently, others have appeared on the market such as Kylie Jenner's Lip Kits. Long-wearing matte lipsticks are popular, but remember, they are a bit drying so take your lip prep seriously.

8 All that's left now is a little setting spray, which you need to be careful when selecting. Many are simply hydrating mists, which can have an adverse effect for those wanting to hold their makeup in place longer. However, Kryolan Fixing Spray and Urban Decay All Nighter are very effective at holding makeup in place.

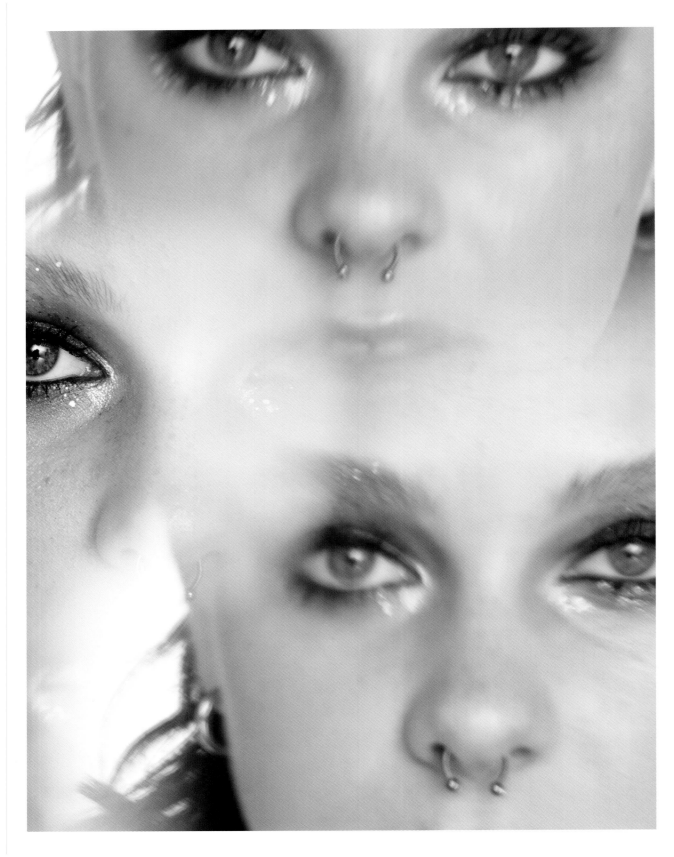

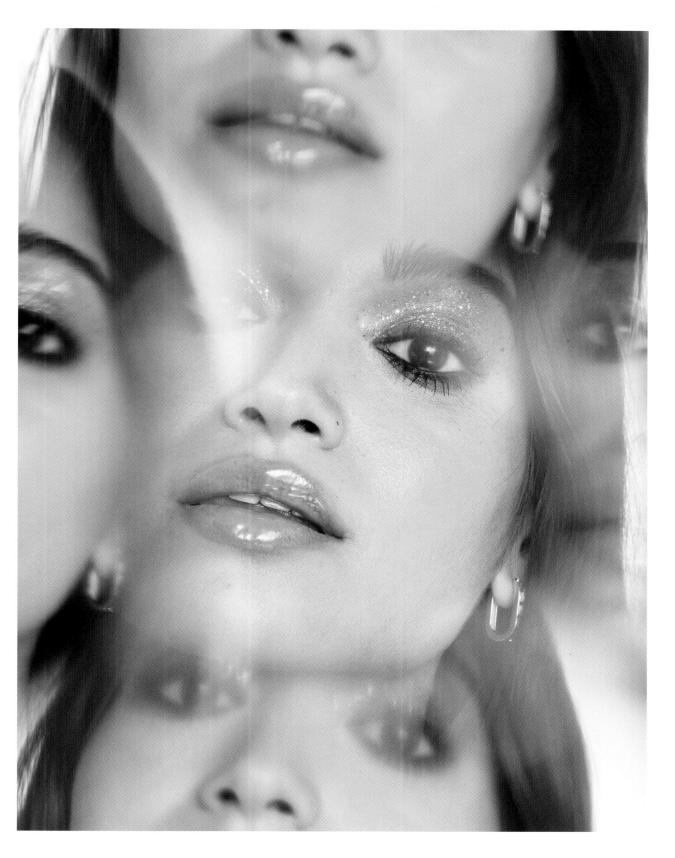

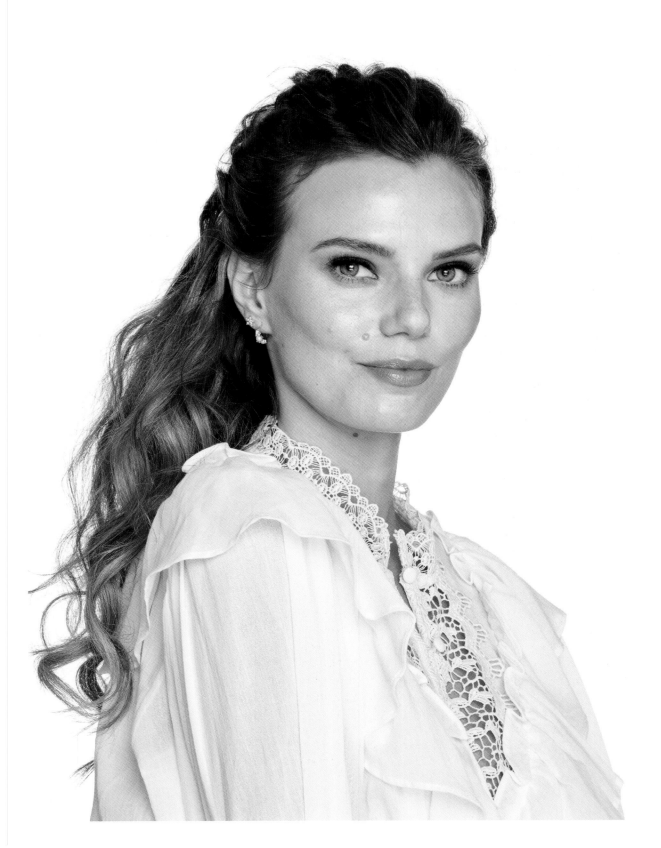

Bridal or Event

I couldn't write a book and not touch on event or bridal makeup. Whilst some may look down on bridal makeup (I know, I don't get it either) I am immensely proud of the work I've done with my brides over the years.

So many of the skills I've learnt and developed working with brides has prepared me for many of the more bizarre, stressful situations I've found myself in. I mean, a wedding morning can feel a bit like backstage at fashion week when you have faces you've never worked on before, a new space to work in that isn't always favourable, limited time, great expectations and heightened emotions, ha!

For years I spent the vast majority of my Saturdays schlepping up and down the country with my ever-growing kit to help get people ready for their big day, often leaving at the crack of dawn to get there in time, often on convoluted train journeys as I'd bought the cheapest possible ticket. It was sometimes even a team effort, as Simon would drive and spend hours in the car park waiting patiently for me to finish. The stories I could tell . . . from being treated like a member of the family to being shouted at by boisterous bridesmaids, it has been a wonderful journey. Some of my brides have even become dear friends, and I still take on brides to this day, simply because I love it so much.

When it comes to makeup for big events, the 'look' is completely subjective, as it should make them feel at their very best. Models are paid for you to make them up however you and your client so wish, but here it is up to the MUA to make their vision come to life, whatever it is.

You should always be your own inspiration. Yes, it can be helpful to tear out images from magazines that you like and screenshot makeup looks that you want to try and replicate but so often when I'm shown images they have little or no resemblance to the person in question – different hair colour, eye colour, skin tone . . . It can therefore be very challenging to replicate the look shown and have the same finish. I always encourage my clients to show me an image of themselves that they feel beautiful in. I know it's not always easy to say 'hey, I think I look good here' but it is helpful to understand what they perceive to be attractive. It is worth noting here that it is much easier to 'see' what you don't like than be able to verbalise what you do like, so don't be afraid to say if there's something you don't like.

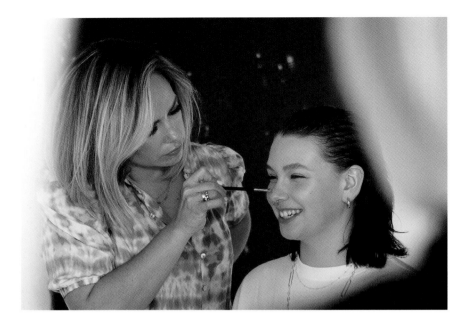

The joy of makeup is that you can tweak it, take it off, add to it – nothing is permanent and a good MUA won't be offended if you want something changed. It should be a collaborative process. There is no 'one size fits all' look, and here are my tips for achieving whatever look you are going for:

I used:

- **Charlotte Tilbury Beautiful Skin Foundation 3 Neutral**
- **Bobbi Brown Light Bisque Corrector**
- **Bobbi Brown Cool Sand Concealer**
- **Charlotte Tilbury Airbrush Powder 01**
- **Mehron Celebre Pro-HD Cream Contour and Highlight Palette**
- **Daniel Sandler Watercolour Blush in So Pretty**
- **Anastasia Beverly Hills Brow Wiz in Soft Brown**
- **Blink Brow Bar Brow Gloss**
- **Charlotte Tilbury Eyes to Mesmerise in Oyster Pearl**
- **Charlotte Tilbury Luxury Eye Palette in Exagger-Eyes**
- **Delilah Gel Liner in Ebony**
- **Bobbi Brown No Smudge Mascara**
- **Sisley Lip Balm**
- **Charlotte Tilbury Pillow Talk Lip Cheat**
- **MAC lipstick in Yash**
- **Clarins Natural Lip Perfector in Toffee Shimmer**
- **Hourglass Ambient Lighting Powder in Luminous Light**
- **Urban Decay All Nighter Setting Spray**

Top tips

1 Focus on skin prep ahead of the day. If you have concerns about your skin, if at all possible visit a dermatologist well in advance for expert guidance. Do not try a miracle treatment or facial close to the day if you haven't had the treatment before. You don't know how your skin will react, so if it's not something you're familiar with, don't do it! The only exception being infrared light therapy, as there is zero risk of reaction but also no dramatic effect either, as it is something that helps over time.

2 Drink a lot of water – it's the best thing for your skin. And I mean unadulterated H_2O. Coffee and tea don't count! I have seen near-miraculous improvements in the skin's overall appearance once water intake is upped.

3 Exfoliate. I do love acids and retinoids, but I advise my clients to exfoliate the night before the big day with a gentle scrub to physically buff off any dead or dry skin cells. I say this because acids and retinoids can leave the skin a little traumatised, maybe not to the naked eye but as soon as you try to put makeup on, the pigments in the makeup can clog in the delicate skin and even the most minuscule flakes look obvious. It's really very tricky to manage and I've been in situations where no amount of moisturiser or oil has been able to fix the problem. A gentle buff with a scrub will be all one needs, always the night before so the skin isn't red or irritated, and so that it can absorb the skincare before bed. You will then wake up with soft, hydrated skin, ready for makeup to sit smoothly on top (once you've cleansed, of course!).

4 Apply a few light layers of your preferred skincare. Don't scrimp on skin prep. Ensuring your skin is well hydrated before makeup will prevent your skin drinking your makeup and going patchy – it will give you the best chance of looking flawless and the makeup lasting all day.

5 Only ever apply SPF under your makeup, not 'in' your foundation or on top of your makeup. SPF can cause 'bounce back' or 'flash back' in flash photography, which can cause a whitish hue in pictures. The titanium dioxide reflects the light and makes a perfect match foundation look significantly paler in photos.

6 Use setting powder. I know lots of people don't like powder and fear it will make their makeup look dry and cakey, but I promise it won't! Just a little through the T-zone and any other area that you secrete oil will really help.

7 Try to mattify hotspots that can look shiny. These are notably the T-zone, just above and in the brows, between the brows and on either side of the nose and the chin.

8 Have a few items on hand for touch-ups: blotting papers, setting powder, blush, lip balm and lipstick. I add blush to the list because there's often a lot of hugging and kissing at events and this can cause makeup to be lifted off the skin. And I list lip balm as there are lots of factors that can contribute to dry lips: nerves, excitement, alcohol and laying lipstick on top of dry lips doesn't look or feel great so I find it's most effective to remove all trace of lip colour, apply balm, blot and then reapply lip colour for the best finish.

These are my top tips if you are doing your own makeup:

1 Practise! The more you practise the more it will feel like second nature. There are so many factors that could potentially cause stress, so you want to eliminate as many as possible – and having your makeup as a slick routine is one of them.

2 Once you've decided on your look, put all the makeup you're going to need in a separate bag, even the night before. On the day you won't then be tempted to use something you haven't worn in ages or get overwhelmed by choice. This happened to me recently when I was getting ready for an awards ceremony. The show I work on was up for an award, so I wanted to look my best. I hadn't planned my look and ended up using a whole load of unusual products and it didn't turn out well. Luckily, we won and I didn't care in the end!

3 Take a picture of yourself when you've finished your makeup to check how it looks. It can be tricky to gauge in the mirror but seeing it in a photo helps. You can then adjust anything accordingly.

4 Do your makeup in an area with good natural light. Spotlights can be particularly tricky to do makeup beneath as they cast shadows over the face, so facing a window can really help.

5 Plan a space for makeup ahead of time. You don't want to feel cramped or stressed.

6 Consider taking yourself away for some alone time to put your makeup on.

7 If you're going to wear fake tan, practise ahead of time so you're prepared for the shade you'll be and colour match your foundation to that.

8 If you are wearing a fake tan, be sure to have it done at least two days before the wedding to allow it to settle. If you get it done the day before it could feel a little strong and you could be left with that fake tan smell. And whatever you do, let the tan dry before putting any clothes on – I've had to try to correct fake tan strap marks and smudges more times than I can count!

9 Don't forget to apply lotion to your body. A good massage with some body moisturiser at least half an hour before getting into your outfit can help you get that ethereal glow.

10 However, if you are using body makeup, DON'T moisturise! To ensure the makeup doesn't transfer onto your outfit, apply the makeup to clean, dry skin, there will be enough moisture in the product to help your skin look its best. If you have particularly dry skin on your body, then be sure to get into a good habit of exfoliating regularly and moisturising after each shower to keep it soft and smooth and hydrated.

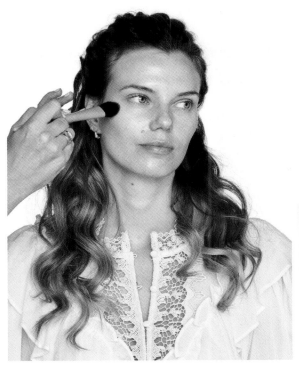

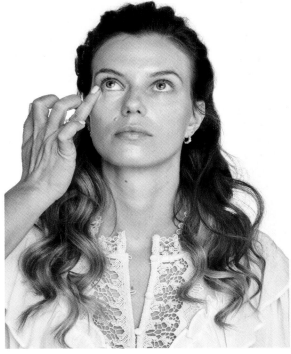

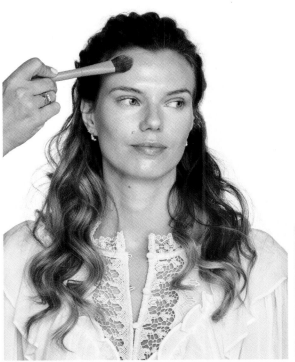

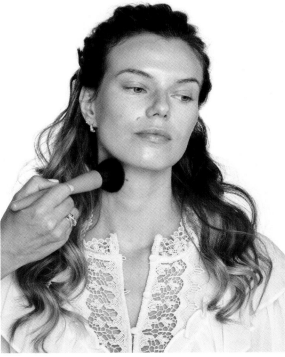

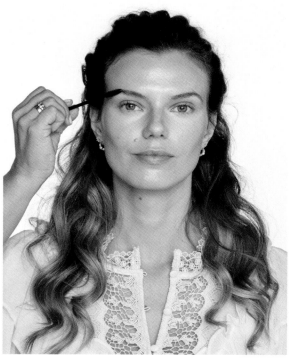

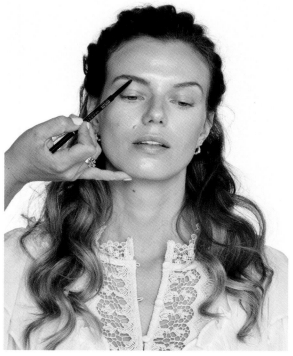

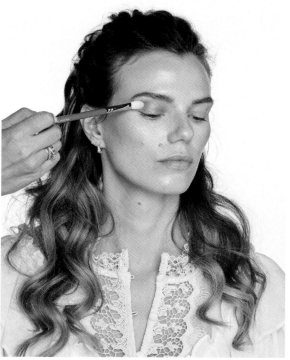

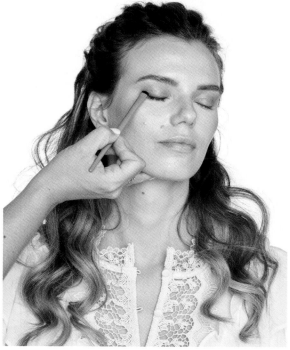

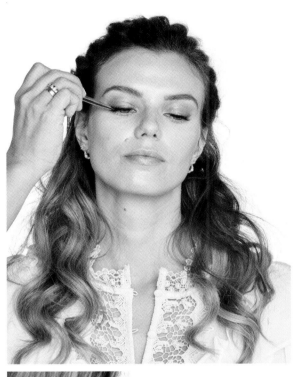
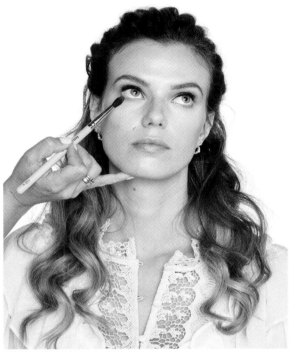
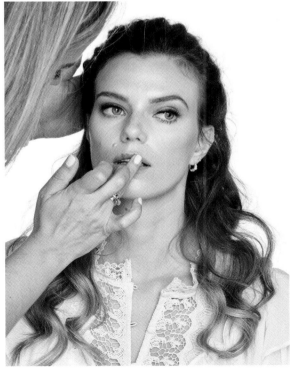
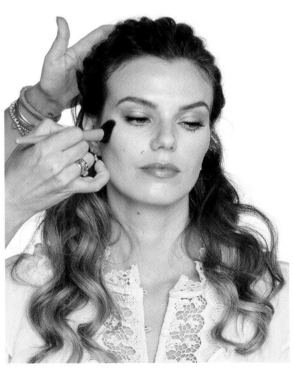

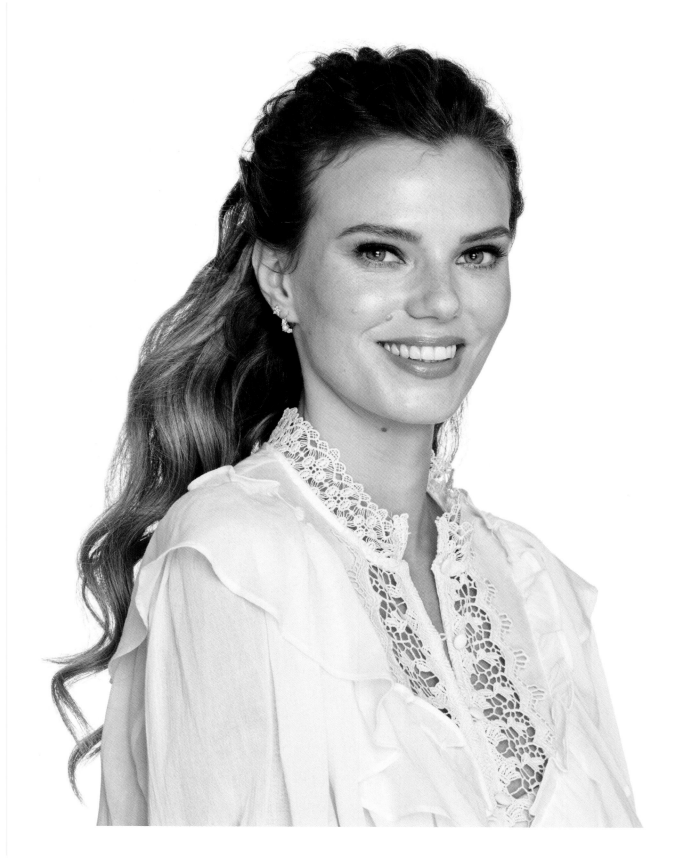

ON THE DAY

A few extra tips that I have learnt, not technically to do with makeup but helpful for prep:

1 To avoid marks, don't wear tight socks or a tight bra on the morning or day of the event.

2 Don't get ready in a top that has to be taken off over your head, to avoid messing up your hair and makeup.

3 Write a schedule and be generous with your timings. I know, that doesn't sound fun or sexy at all, but it really helps to make sure everything runs to time. There's nothing worse than feeling stressed and running late.

4 Eat and stay hydrated. You need to keep your energy up and keep headaches at bay.

5 Wear your shoes in to avoid getting blisters. If you're worried about scuffing your shoes, put them in a plastic bag and walk around in them! Score the sole so that you don't slip.

6 Carry a handkerchief. If you do cry and dab with a tissue, then the tissue can disintegrate and get stuck in your makeup (or, even worse, get in your eye) so carry a hankie that you can delicately dab to absorb any tears. Don't wipe. Wiping could move your makeup. If you do think you're about to cry and don't want to, inhale deeply through your nose, repeatedly, if necessary, and it sometimes helps prevent those threatening tears from rolling down the cheek.

7 Carry mints. Nerves, anxiety, excitement, dehydration and alcohol can lead to stale breath, so have mints handy to freshen your breath and reactive your saliva glands.

8 Carry a little perfume. Just like touching up your blush and lipstick, a refresh of your fragrance can be really uplifting.

Holiday Makeup

I've never been one to pack lightly for holiday! Mainly because it's often on holiday that I have a little more time to enjoy the process of putting on makeup, unlike at home where I'm often slapping it on to rush out of the door! However, I'm frequently asked for help from those wanting to streamline their makeup bag with items that will stand up in warm conditions, so see below my list of 10 holiday makeup essentials:

1 **SPF** – I swear by the Sun Bum SPF 50 Spray for the body as it's not sticky, smells amazing and gets zero resistance from the kids! The La Roche-Posay Anthelios SPF 50 Spray is excellent too. For my face I love the Shiseido Clear Suncare Stick SPF 50. So easy to apply, non-sticky, less messy or greasy feeling than creams and great under makeup.

2 **Concealer** – A little something to dab under the eyes and possibly over the cheeks. I love my L'Oréal Infallible concealer or my Bobbi Brown Skin Concealer Stick if you want something a little lighter in texture. I love the latter as a light base instead of foundation and the stick format is small and compact, perfect for travel . . .

3 **Tinted Moisturiser** – This is optional in my opinion. If you have a concealer you don't necessarily need another base product, but for those who usually wear foundation and want some kind of base then a tint is great on holiday. Two I love are the Laura Mercier Tinted Moisturiser and the Rimmel Kind and Free Moisturising Skin Tint Foundation. If you're going somewhere particularly humid you may wish to choose the oil-free version of the Laura Mercier.

4 **Blotting Paper** – Light, compact, portable and excellent for mattifying the skin and absorbing both oil and perspiration. I prefer this option to powder when I'm on holiday but if you're a powder lover at heart then the Huda Beauty Baby Bake Loose Setting Powder Mini is fantastic.

5 **Bronzer** – Of course I'm going to recommend bronzer as it is the ultimate in skin-rejuvenating colour! Gels and sticks are great space savers. For gels, I recommend the Iconic London Sheer Bronze, Clinique Sun-Kissed Face Gelee. For sticks, I love the Rare Beauty Warm Wishes Effortless Bronzer, Nudestix Nudies and Pixi On-the-Glow Bronze. If you want a highlighting stick then the Ciaté Dewy Stix Bronzing Balm is the best.

6 **Blush Stick** – Small and portable, I recommend a blush stick for holiday packing but also because they add that enviable glow to the cheeks. The Nudestix Nudies Blush Sticks are my go-to as there are lots of shade choice and both matte and shimmer formulas. The Huda Beauty Cheeky Tint Blush Sticks, Revolution Fast Base Blush Sticks, Clinique Chubby Sticks, Anastasia Beverly Hills Stick Blush and Jones Road Lip and Cheek Sticks are great too. They can be used on eyes, lips and cheeks, so are super versatile!

7 **Brows** – My brows and curling my lashes is sometimes all I do when heading for a day at the beach. The Benefit Precisely, My Brow and Makeup Forever Aqua Resist Brow Definer are excellent and clear gels work well in water and heat, so something like the Blink Brow Bar Clear Gloss or Anastasia Beverly Hills Clear Brow Gel would be great.

8 **Long-wear Cream Shadow Sticks** – These are brilliant not least because they're small and portable, but also because once they are applied they do not budge! The OG is the Bobbi Brown Long Wear Cream Shadow Stick but Beauty Pie also make excellent ones as do Laura Mercier, Trish McEvoy, Vieve, Kiko Milano and NYX.

9 **Mascara** – Tubing or waterproof is essential to avoid smudging around the eyes if you go for a swim or are in warm and sticky conditions. My favourite tubing mascara is the Trish McEvoy High Volume Tubular Mascara and for waterproof I swear by the Bobbi Brown No Smudge Mascara, Clinique High Impact Waterproof Mascara and both Lancôme's Idole and Hypnôse Waterproof mascaras.

10 **Lip Balm/Lipstick** – Lip balm with an SPF is a must on holiday. I'm a sucker for the Bondi Sands and Sun Bum lip balms, although the Nivea Lip SPF 30 and Revolution Lip Protector SPF 30 are also very good.

'YOU ASKED'

You Asked

Can anyone wear a smokey eye?

Absolutely, yes! You can have fun blending multiple shades or you can keep it simple by sweeping a single muted shadow all over the eyelid, blending the edges and smudging along the lower lash line. Finish with lashings of mascara. Colour-wise, I recommend Mocha, Pewter, Copper, Bronze, and Charcoal tones.

Are primers essential?

In my opinion, no. It's a misconception that they will set your makeup in place for the day. They can be useful, but I prefer to concentrate on a simple skincare routine that meets your skins needs. This is the best way to prep your skin before applying makeup.

How do I know if I'm wearing the right shade of foundation?

Most simply: you'll know you've got the right colour if you can't see the shade on your skin. It is always best to test the foundation through the centre of the face and if it disappears with very little blending then you're on to a good thing!

How do I prevent getting mascara on my top lid?

There are tools that you can buy to place behind your top lashes to prevent any mascara from transferring onto your eyelids. But I always recommend that you tilt your head back and look down into a mirror to create space between your lash line and your lid.

If I have SPF in my foundation, do I still need to wear a separate SPF under my makeup?

Yes! Whilst SPF in foundation provides some protection, you'd need to use a lot of foundation to get the full SPF protection they offer. I recommend using dedicated sun protection every day before you apply your makeup.

Will makeup clog my pores?

Makeup technology has advanced so much in the last 100 years. As long as you remove makeup thoroughly every night by double cleansing, your pores won't clog. If you're particularly concerned about clogged pores, look for products that are non-comedogenic.

Is there such a thing as the perfect red lip?

I believe so, in that if you love a particular shade, then you should keep wearing it and just enjoy yourself! Don't worry too much about 'the rules' when it comes to reds. However, if you're not sure or want to try a red lip for the first time, a useful guide is that those with fair skin tend to suit cooler reds with a hint of pink; olive skin tones suit orangey reds; and black and brown skin tones look stunning in bold, rich, deep reds. But honestly, if you love the colour, just wear it with confidence.

How long should makeup last?

You can find this out by looking at your makeup packaging. On the box, you will find a small image of a pot with a number beside it. This number advises on how many months the makeup will remain good for use once it has been opened (e.g.: 6M = 6 months, 12M = 12 months, 24M = 24 months etc.). It is particularly important to follow these guidelines when it comes to skincare, as 'clean' formulas can go off quickly and some actives cease being affective after time. When it comes to powder makeup, scrape the surface off and spray with antibacterial makeup spray to preserve the shelf life.

I'm in my 60's – am I too old to wear glitter?

Absolutely not! Glitter is for anyone and everyone who loves a bit of sparkle. The finer the glitter, the more flattering it will be.

I'm always in a rush in the mornings. How long should it take me to do my makeup?

How long is a piece of string?! I love nothing more than a chilled, indulgent makeup moment, but you can absolutely do a decent version of everyday makeup in under 5 minutes. If you need inspiration, I have lots of 5-minute makeup routines on my Instagram (@hannahmartinmakeup) as well as a step-by-step guide to creating the look on page 229.

Why does my concealer always crease?

Concealer can crease under the eye because most of us have very fine lines in this area. To avoid this, add only a little eye cream to the area before makeup application and take some time to gently work the concealer into the skin (I like to press mine into place with the pad of my ring finger). Set with a little loose powder, and this should prevent concealer from creasing too much.

My lipstick comes off within minutes of applying it. How can I avoid this?

Some lipsticks are made to be more long lasting than others. Balm-based lipsticks and those that claim to be hydrating generally won't last as long as a matte lipstick. However, there are now lots of liquid lipsticks available that wear extremely well. If you want to extend the wear of a lipstick you already have, then use a lip pencil to fill in the entire lip – this will give your lipstick something to adhere to. Apply your lipstick over the top, blot with a tissue, set with a little loose powder (push through a single ply of tissue held over the lips) then apply the lipstick colour again to set.

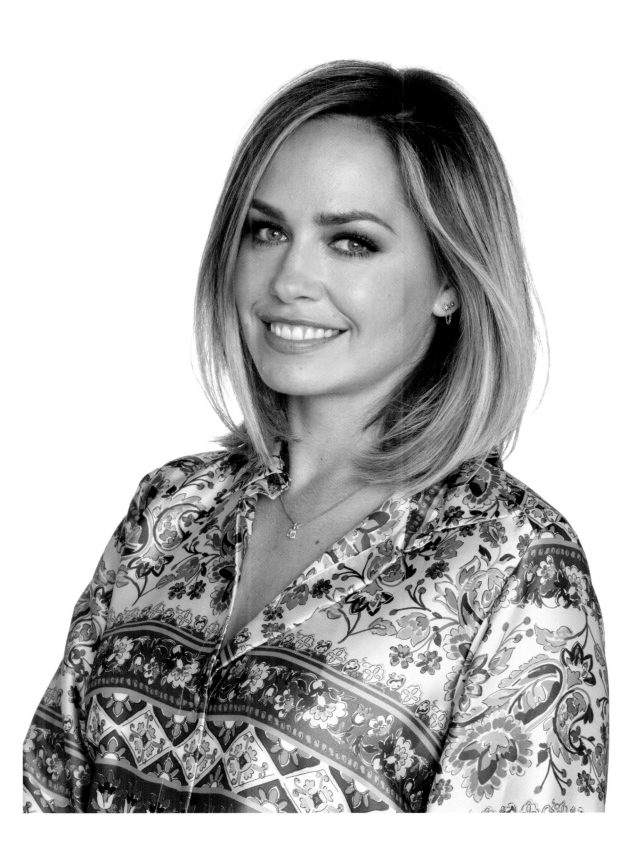

Index

Acknowledgements

Where to start with all my very many thank yous!

It's taken a small village to get this book written but I wouldn't even be writing it if it wasn't for you Bev, Aoife, Tom and everyone at Bev James Management. I can't thank you enough for believing in me when I didn't believe in myself. The girl who gave up on her dissertation has only gone and done it! Goes to show what you can achieve when you have the right people behind you. Aoife in particular – thank you for keeping on top of it all and collating my many reems of ramblings – who knew I could write a book on a laptop I can barely navigate? Everyone writes their books in Notes right? Honestly, you're such an integral cog in this machine. I am eternally grateful for all your support.

To Louise and everyone at HarperCollins and HQ. Your excitement and enthusiasm for this book has kept me going – thank you for being on board with all my ideas and bringing them to life. Dreams coming true right here. Louise, thank you for taking my words and ordering them in a way that makes sense.

To the book shoot crew – thank you – we did it! To my amazing photographers: Sarah, it just had to be you, you're the best in beauty, thank you. To Amelia, one of my besties and renowned food photographer, thank you for coming on board and agreeing to photograph the products for me, another fun thing to add to a lifetime of hilarious adventures . . . Charlie, Charlie . . . (it's a pj!)!

To Lewis – thank you for your hair genius and for almost behaving, love ya.

To my makeup assistants Jess and Zara – I love you both so much, there's no one I'd rather have on set with me. Thank you.

To my models. I'll start with you, Sue, my wonderful mother-in-law. Who knew you could start a modelling career just shy of 70! Thank you for agreeing to be in my book and for allowing Lewis to change your parting. Your heart radiates in your pictures and you look absolutely beautiful. Arlo. What can I say? You're family to me and my family. I'm so grateful you agreed to let me do your makeup and be photographed, again. I'm here for you always, no matter what. To Jessica, thank you for your friendship and for bringing all your stunning Scream Pretty jewellery to dress the models for the shoot. I'm delighted we got you in front of the camera, you beautiful creature. And Zara. That smile! Thank you for agreeing to tackle my colour challenge and taking a moment on set – you're just gorgeous inside and out – love you. Huge thank you to the actual models Kiera, Desiree, Raihanna and Eilie.

To all those who've been instrumental in my career as a makeup artist. Melissa Heyward-Fisher you were the first to take a chance on the then miserable nursing student and gave me my first makeup job at Benefit. Those days in Debenhams Oxford, although not for long, are some of my fondest memories – Sally, Sharon, Abby, Helen, Nimi et al.

Sarah Jamieson – I'm so grateful you gave me my first job at Bobbi Brown Cosmetics. Thank you for not writing me off as a weirdo after I called you daily until you agreed to meet with me. That interview in Starbucks South Molton Street will go down in history as a pivotal moment for me.

From the retail days in HOF City (Roxy, Lisa, Stephanie, Liz, Sevda – you guys made work such a pleasure) and Fenwick Bond St (Neria, Louisa, Layla) until I stepped out of store and into the Pro Team. Thank you, Paul, George, Nikki, Alberto, those were the good old days eh! Good times but also some of my darkest days personally . . . To the brand managers that so inspired me – Cheryl and Quita – but it was you, Bethan Williams, who first gave me the notion I could be more than just a counter manager. It was the time you spoke to us central London studio managers in the Grosvenor St training room and told us you were looking at future Brand Directors. I'd never even considered at that point that that could be the case but my goodness I've never forgotten it.

Then to Bobbi Brown herself. From meeting you that first time at the Ham Yard Hotel in 2007, I never dreamed that I'd one day be a part of your team but I thank you from the bottom of my heart for EVERYTHING. Your love, support, friendship and mentorship, the opportunities you've given me, the doors you've opened both whilst at your brand and since – there aren't enough words to express my gratitude.

Krishna Montgomery, yes, you. You were the one who gave me that final nudge I needed to step out on my own. THANK YOU for holding my hand that first year, it's thanks to you that we secured *10 Years Younger* and thanks to that that I have my very own NRTA Award for Best Fashion and Makeup show. On that note, thank you Nicole for casting me. Taping that screen test in my kitchen was one of the most surreal moments of my life! Ha! To the *10YY* Glam team- John, Gemma, Tapan, Nilam and Uchenna, I love you guys.

Marcia – that DM the day I announced I was going solo gave me such hope that there were opportunities waiting for me.

To my makeup agents past and present – Helen and Lindsay at Premier and Claire at 18 Management, thank you for keeping my makeup work alive when my schedule is so busy.

To my clients, I won't name you but you know who you are. Thank you for entrusting me with your faces for some of the key moments in your life – I love you all and your crews so much.

To the brands, PR agencies and retailers who have entrusted me to share their vision and educate through social media, I thank you for choosing me.

To all of the beauty editors and beauty press who have been so supportive and featured my work on their pages and online, thank you!

A special shout out to Charlotte and the entire team at Ciaté – who knew that first gig launching your Wonderful Skin Foundation would lead to where we are now. A sell-out edit and our stunning brush collection. Thank you, thank you for saying yes!

And to my most important team of all. My family. Pops and Noodle, Rob and Sue, my darling Sal. The friends who have become family: Amelia, Alice, Annabelle, Harriet, Rachel, Sarah, Sara. The 'Holy Hoes' – an ironic name for a group of women who met at church! The mums who keep me sane and caffeinated: Mailika, Nim and Lorraine. Jane – you're known as 'Legend' in our house for a reason – without your help we'd be a hot mess. But the biggest thanks of all goes to you my darling Simon and our children Bear and Bo. I couldn't do any of this without you and I wouldn't want to. You guys ALWAYS come first and I love you with all my heart.

HQ
An imprint of HarperCollins*Publishers* Ltd
1 London Bridge Street
London SE1 9GF

www.harpercollins.co.uk

HarperCollins*Publishers*
Macken House, 39/40 Mayor Street Upper
Dublin 1
D01 C9W8 Ireland

10 9 8 7 6 5 4 3 2

First published in Great Britain by
HQ, an imprint of HarperCollins*Publishers* Ltd 2023

ISBN 978-0-00-850442-7

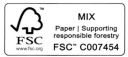

This book is produced from independently certified FSC™ paper to ensure
responsible forest management.

For more information visit:
www.harpercollins.co.uk/green

Printed and bound in Bosnia and Herzegovina by GPS Group

Design: Louise Evans
Model photography: Sarah Brown
Product and BTS photography: Amelia Johnson
Models: Arlo, Desiree @ Zone Models, Eilie @ MOT Models, Jessica, Kira
 @ Zone Models, Lewis, Raihanna @ MOT Models, Sue, Zara
Makeup: Hannah Martin
Makeup Assistants: Jessica Doyle and Zara Findlay
Hair: Lewis Palett
Jewellery: Scream Pretty
Nails: Jessica Thompson
Editorial Director: Louise McKeever
Production: Halema Begum

Model photography
© Sarah Brown 2023

Product and behind-the-scenes
photography
© Amelia Johnson 2023

Images on pages 14–15 and 78
© Hannah Martin 2023

Images on pages 101 and 145
and makeup effects
© Shutterstock 2023

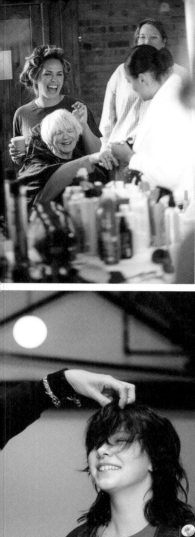
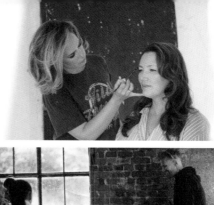
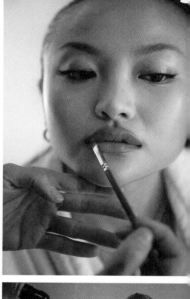
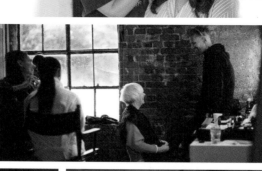
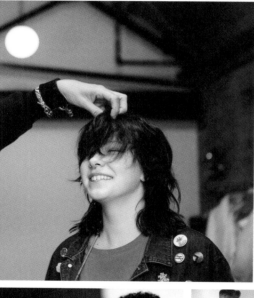
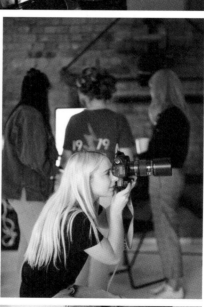
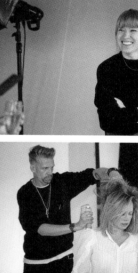
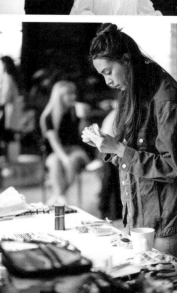
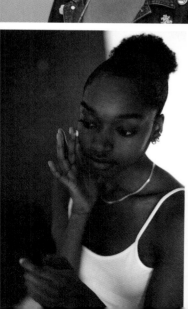
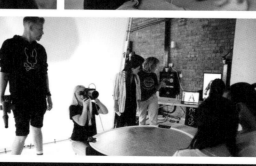
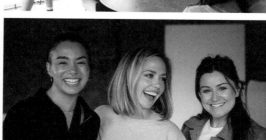